Handbook of Functional MRI Data Analysis

Functional magnetic resonance imaging (fMRI) has become the most popular method for imaging brain function. *Handbook of Functional MRI Data Analysis* provides a comprehensive and practical introduction to the methods used for fMRI data analysis. Using minimal jargon, this book explains the concepts behind processing fMRI data, focusing on the techniques that are most commonly used in the field. This book provides background about the methods employed by common data analysis packages including FSL, SPM, and AFNI. Some of the newest cutting-edge techniques, including pattern classification analysis, connectivity modeling, and resting state network analysis, are also discussed.

Readers of this book, whether newcomers to the field or experienced researchers, will obtain a deep and effective knowledge of how to employ fMRI analysis to ask scientific questions and become more sophisticated users of fMRI analysis software.

Dr. Russell A. Poldrack is the director of the Imaging Research Center and professor of Psychology and Neurobiology at the University of Texas at Austin. He has published more than 100 articles in the field of cognitive neuroscience, in journals including *Science, Nature, Neuron, Nature Neuroscience*, and *PNAS*. He is well known for his writings on how neuroimaging can be used to make inferences about psychological function, as well as for his research using fMRI and other imaging techniques to understand the brain systems that support learning and memory, decision making, and executive function.

Dr. Jeanette A. Mumford is a research assistant professor in the Department of Psychology at the University of Texas at Austin. Trained in biostatistics, her research has focused on the development and characterization of new methods for statistical modeling and analysis of fMRI data. Her work has examined the impact of different group modeling strategies and developed new tools for modeling network structure in resting-state fMRI data. She is the developer of the fmriPower software package, which provides power analysis tools for fMRI data.

Dr. Thomas E. Nichols is the head of Neuroimaging Statistics at the University of Warwick, United Kingdom. He has been working in functional neuroimaging since 1992, when he joined the University of Pittsburgh's PET facility as programmer and statistician. He is known for his work on inference in brain imaging, using both parametric and nonparametric methods, and he is an active contributor to the FSL and SPM software packages. In 2009 he received the Wiley Young Investigator Award from the Organization for Human Brain Mapping in recognition for his contributions to statistical modeling and inference of neuroimaging data.

Handbook of Functional MRI Data Analysis

Russell A. Poldrack
University of Texas at Austin, Imaging Research Center

Jeanette A. Mumford
University of Texas at Austin

Thomas E. Nichols
University of Warwick

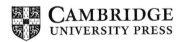
CAMBRIDGE
UNIVERSITY PRESS

CAMBRIDGE UNIVERSITY PRESS
Cambridge, New York, Melbourne, Madrid, Cape Town,
Singapore, São Paulo, Delhi, Mexico City

Cambridge University Press
32 Avenue of the Americas, New York, NY 10013-2473, USA

www.cambridge.org
Information on this title: www.cambridge.org/9780521517669

First published 2011
Reprinted 2012 (twice)

Printed in the United States of America

A catalog record for this publication is available from the British Library.

Library of Congress Cataloging in Publication Data

Poldrack, Russell A.
    Handbook of functional MRI data analysis / Russell A. Poldrack,
    Jeanette A. Mumford, Thomas E. Nichols.
        p. ; cm.
    Includes bibliographical references and index.
    ISBN 978-0-521-51766-9 (hardback)
    1. Brain mapping – Statistical methods. 2. Brain – Imaging – Statistical methods.
    3. Magnetic resonance imaging. I. Mumford, Jeanette A., 1975–
    II. Nichols, Thomas E. III. Title.
    [DNLM: 1. Magnetic Resonance Imaging. 2. Brain Mapping. 3. Data Interpretation,
    Statistical. 4. Image Processing, Computer-Assisted – methods. WN 185]
    RC386.6.B7P65 2011
    616.8′047548–dc22   2011010349

ISBN 978-0-521-51766-9 Hardback

Contents

Preface   *page* ix

1   Introduction   1
     1.1   A brief overview of fMRI   1
     1.2   The emergence of cognitive neuroscience   3
     1.3   A brief history of fMRI analysis   4
     1.4   Major components of fMRI analysis   7
     1.5   Software packages for fMRI analysis   7
     1.6   Choosing a software package   10
     1.7   Overview of processing streams   10
     1.8   Prerequisites for fMRI analysis   10

2   Image processing basics   13
     2.1   What is an image?   13
     2.2   Coordinate systems   15
     2.3   Spatial transformations   17
     2.4   Filtering and Fourier analysis   31

3   Preprocessing fMRI data   34
     3.1   Introduction   34
     3.2   An overview of fMRI preprocessing   34
     3.3   Quality control techniques   34
     3.4   Distortion correction   38
     3.5   Slice timing correction   41
     3.6   Motion correction   43
     3.7   Spatial smoothing   50

4   Spatial normalization   53
     4.1   Introduction   53
     4.2   Anatomical variability   53
     4.3   Coordinate spaces for neuroimaging   54

4.4	Atlases and templates	55
4.5	Preprocessing of anatomical images	56
4.6	Processing streams for fMRI normalization	58
4.7	Spatial normalization methods	60
4.8	Surface-based methods	62
4.9	Choosing a spatial normalization method	63
4.10	Quality control for spatial normalization	65
4.11	Troubleshooting normalization problems	66
4.12	Normalizing data from special populations	66
5	**Statistical modeling: Single subject analysis**	70
5.1	The BOLD signal	70
5.2	The BOLD noise	86
5.3	Study design and modeling strategies	92
6	**Statistical modeling: Group analysis**	100
6.1	The mixed effects model	100
6.2	Mean centering continuous covariates	105
7	**Statistical inference on images**	110
7.1	Basics of statistical inference	110
7.2	Features of interest in images	112
7.3	The multiple testing problem and solutions	116
7.4	Combining inferences: masking and conjunctions	123
7.5	Use of region of interest masks	126
7.6	Computing statistical power	126
8	**Modeling brain connectivity**	130
8.1	Introduction	130
8.2	Functional connectivity	131
8.3	Effective connectivity	144
8.4	Network analysis and graph theory	155
9	**Multivoxel pattern analysis and machine learning**	160
9.1	Introduction to pattern classification	160
9.2	Applying classifiers to fMRI data	163
9.3	Data extraction	163
9.4	Feature selection	164
9.5	Training and testing the classifier	165
9.6	Characterizing the classifier	171
10	**Visualizing, localizing, and reporting fMRI data**	173
10.1	Visualizing activation data	173
10.2	Localizing activation	176

10.3 Localizing and reporting activation   179
10.4 Region of interest analysis   183

Appendix A   Review of the General Linear Model   191
    A.1 Estimating GLM parameters   191
    A.2 Hypothesis testing   194
    A.3 Correlation and heterogeneous variances   195
    A.4 Why "general" linear model?   197

Appendix B   Data organization and management   201
    B.1 Computing for fMRI analysis   201
    B.2 Data organization   202
    B.3 Project management   204
    B.4 Scripting for data analysis   205

Appendix C   Image formats   208
    C.1 Data storage   208
    C.2 File formats   209

Bibliography   211
Index   225

Preface

Functional magnetic resonance imaging (fMRI) has, in less than two decades, become the most commonly used method for the study of human brain function. FMRI is a technique that uses magnetic resonance imaging to measure brain activity by measuring changes in the local oxygenation of blood, which in turn reflects the amount of local brain activity. The analysis of fMRI data is exceedingly complex, requiring the use of sophisticated techniques from signal and image processing and statistics in order to go from the raw data to the finished product, which is generally a statistical map showing which brain regions responded to some particular manipulation of mental or perceptual functions. There are now several software packages available for the processing and analysis of fMRI data, several of which are freely available.

The purpose of this book is to provide researchers with a sophisticated understanding of all of the techniques necessary for processing and analysis of fMRI data. The content is organized roughly in line with the standard flow of data processing operations, or processing stream, used in fMRI data analysis. After starting with a general introduction to fMRI, the chapters walk through all the steps that one takes in analyzing an fMRI dataset. We begin with an overview of basic image processing methods, providing an introduction to the kinds of data that are used in fMRI and how they can be transformed and filtered. We then discuss the many steps that are used for preprocessing fMRI data, including quality control, correction for various kinds of artifacts, and spatial smoothing, followed by a description of methods for spatial normalization, which is the warping of data into a common anatomical space. The next three chapters then discuss the heart of fMRI data analysis, which is statistical modeling and inference. We separately discuss modeling data from fMRI timeseries within an individual and modeling group data across individuals, followed by an outline of methods for statistical inference that focuses on the severe multiple test problem that is inherent in fMRI data. Two additional chapters focus on methods for analyzing data that go beyond a single voxel, involving either the modeling of connectivity between regions or the use of machine learning techniques to model multivariate patterns in the data. The final chapter discusses approaches for the visualization of the complex data that come out of fMRI analysis. The appendices provide background about the general linear model, a practical guide to the organization of fMRI data, and an introduction to imaging data file formats.

The intended audience for this book is individuals who want to understand fMRI analysis at a deep conceptual level, rather than simply knowing which buttons to push on the software package. This may include graduate students and advanced undergraduate students, medical school students, and researchers in a broad range of fields including psychology, neuroscience, radiology, neurology, statistics, and bioinformatics. The book could be used in a number of types of courses, including graduate and advanced undergraduate courses on neuroimaging as well as more focused courses on fMRI data analysis.

We have attempted to explain the concepts in this book with a minimal amount of mathematical notation. Some of the chapters include mathematical detail about particular techniques, but this can generally be skipped without harm, though interested readers will find that understanding the mathematics can provide additional insight. The reader is assumed to have a basic knowledge of statistics and linear algebra, but we also provide background for the reader in these topics, particularly with regard to the general linear model.

We believe that the only way to really learn about fMRI analysis is to do it. To that end, we have provided the example datasets used in the book along with example analysis scripts on the book's Web site: http://www.fmri-data-analysis.org/.

Although our examples focus primarily on the FSL and SPM software packages, we welcome developers and users of other packages to submit example scripts that demonstrate how to analyze the data using those other packages. Another great way to learn about fMRI analysis is to simulate data and test out different techniques. To assist the reader in this exercise, we also provide on the Web site examples of code that was used to create a number of the figures in the book. These examples include MATLAB, R, and Python code, highlighting the many different ways in which one can work with fMRI data.

The following people provided helpful comments on various chapters in the book, for which we are very grateful: Akram Bakkour, Michael Chee, Joe Devlin, Marta Garrido, Clark Glymour, Yaroslav Halchenko, Mark Jenkinson, Agatha Lenartowicz, Randy McIntosh, Rajeev Raizada, Antonio Rangel, David Schnyer, and Klaas Enno Stephan. We would also like to thank Lauren Cowles at Cambridge University Press for her guidance and patience throughout the process of creating this book.

Introduction

The goal of this book is to provide the reader with a solid background in the techniques used for processing and analysis of functional magnetic resonance imaging (fMRI) data.

1.1 A brief overview of fMRI

Since its development in the early 1990s, fMRI has taken the scientific world by storm. This growth is easy to see from the plot of the number of papers that mention the technique in the PubMed database of biomedical literature, shown in Figure 1.1. Back in 1996 it was possible to sit down and read the entirety of the fMRI literature in a week, whereas now it is barely feasible to read all of the fMRI papers that were published in the previous week! The reason for this explosion in interest is that fMRI provides an unprecedented ability to safely and noninvasively image brain activity with very good spatial resolution and relatively good temporal resolution compared to previous methods such as positron emission tomography (PET).

1.1.1 Blood flow and neuronal activity

The most common method of fMRI takes advantage of the fact that when neurons in the brain become active, the amount of blood flowing through that area is increased. This phenomenon has been known for more than 100 years, though the mechanisms that cause it remain only partly understood. What is particularly interesting is that the amount of blood that is sent to the area is more than is needed to replenish the oxygen that is used by the activity of the cells. Thus, the activity-related increase in blood flow caused by neuronal activity leads to a relative surplus in local blood oxygen. The signal measured in fMRI depends on this change in oxygenation and is referred to as the blood oxygenation level dependent, or BOLD, signal.

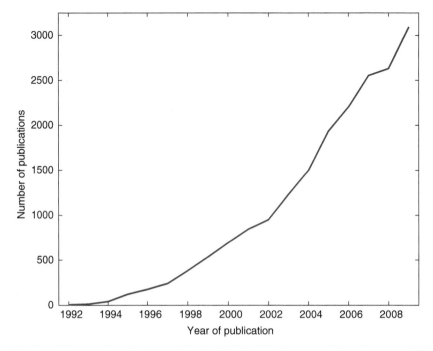

Figure 1.1.   A plot of the number of citations in the PubMed database matching the query ["fMRI" OR "functional MRI" OR "functional magnetic resonance imaging"] for every year since 1992.

Figure 1.2 shows an example of what is known as the *hemodynamic response*, which is the increase in blood flow that follows a brief period of neuronal activity. There are two facts about the hemodynamic response that underlie the basic features of BOLD fMRI and determine how the data must be analyzed. First, the hemodynamic response is slow; whereas neuronal activity may only last milliseconds, the increase in blood flow that follows this activity takes about 5 seconds to reach its maximum. This peak is followed by a long undershoot that does not fully return to baseline for at least 15–20 seconds. Second, the hemodynamic response can, to a first approximation, be treated as a *linear time-invariant* system (Cohen, 1997; Boynton et al., 1996; Dale, 1999). This topic will be discussed in much greater detail in Chapter 5, but in essence the idea is that the response to a long train of neuronal activity can be determined by adding together shifted versions of the response to a shorter train of activity. This linearity makes it possible to create a straightforward statistical model that describes the timecourse of hemodynamic signals that would be expected given some particular timecourse of neuronal activity, using the mathematical operation of *convolution*.

1.1.2 Magnetic resonance imaging

The incredible capabilities of magnetic resonance imaging (MRI) can hardly be overstated. In less than 10 minutes, it is possible to obtain images of the human

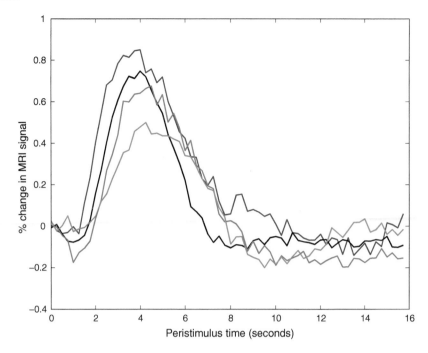

Figure 1.2.   An example of the hemodynamic responses evoked in area V1 by a contrast-reversing checkerboard displayed for 500 ms. The four different lines are data from four different individuals, showing how variable these responses can be across people. The MRI signal was measured every 250 ms, which accounts for the noisiness of the plots. (Data courtesy of Stephen Engel, University of Minnesota)

brain that rival the quality of a postmortem examination, in a completely safe and noninvasive way. Before the development of MRI, imaging primarily relied upon the use of ionizing radiation (as used in X-rays, computed tomography, and positron emission tomography). In addition to the safety concerns about radiation, none of these techniques could provide the flexibility to image the broad range of tissue characteristics that can be measured with MRI. Thus, the establishment of MRI as a standard medical imaging tool in the 1980s led to a revolution in the ability to see inside the human body.

1.2 The emergence of cognitive neuroscience

Our fascination with how the brain and mind are related is about as old as humanity itself. Until the development of neuroimaging methods, the only way to understand how mental function is organized in the brain was to examine the brains of individuals who had suffered damage due to stroke, infection, or injury. It was through these kinds of studies that many early discoveries were made about the localization of mental functions in the brain (though many of these have come into question subsequently). However, progress was limited by the many difficulties that arise in studying brain-damaged patients (Shallice, 1988).

In order to better understand how mental functions relate to brain processes in the normal state, researchers needed a way to image brain function while individuals performed mental tasks designed to manipulate specific mental processes. In the 1980s several groups of researchers (principally at Washington University in St. Louis and the Karolinska Institute in Sweden) began to use positron emission tomography (PET) to ask these questions. PET measures the breakdown of radioactive materials within the body. By using radioactive tracers that are attached to biologically important molecules (such as water or glucose), it can measure aspects of brain function such as blood flow or glucose metabolism. PET showed that it was possible to localize mental functions in the brain, providing the first glimpses into the neural organization of cognition in normal individuals (e.g., Posner et al., 1988). However, the use of PET was limited due to safety concerns about radiation exposure, and due to the scarce availability of PET systems.

fMRI provided exactly the tool that cognitive neuroscience was looking for. First, it was safe, which meant that it could be used in a broad range of individuals, who could be scanned repeatedly many times if necessary. It could also be used with children, who could not take part in PET studies unless the scan was medically necessary. Second, by the 1990s MRI systems had proliferated, such that nearly every medical center had at least one scanner and often several. Because fMRI could be performed on many standard MRI scanners (and today on nearly all of them), it was accessible to many more researchers than PET had been. Finally, fMRI had some important technical benefits over PET. In particular, its spatial resolution (i.e., its ability to resolve small structures) was vastly better than PET. In addition, whereas PET required scans lasting at least a minute, with fMRI it was possible to examine events happening much more quickly. Cognitive neuroscientists around the world quickly jumped on the bandwagon, and thus the growth spurt of fMRI began.

1.3 A brief history of fMRI analysis

When the first fMRI researchers collected their data in the early 1990s, they also had to create the tools to analyze the data, as there was no "off-the-shelf" software for analysis of fMRI data. The first experimental designs and analytic approaches were inspired by analysis of blood flow data using PET. In PET blood flow studies, acquisition of each image takes at least one minute, and a single task is repeated for the entire acquisition. The individual images are then compared using simple statistical procedures such as a t-test between task and resting images. Inspired by this approach, early studies created activation maps by simply subtracting the average activation during one task from activation during another. For example, in the study by Kwong et al. (1992), blocks of visual stimulation were alternated with blocks of no stimulation. As shown in Figure 1.3, the changes in signal in the visual cortex

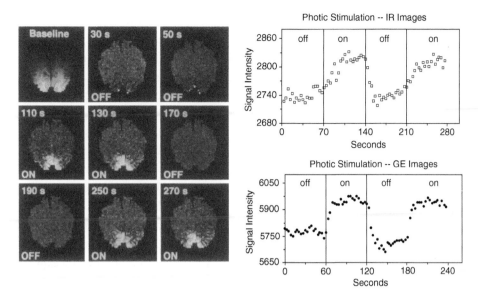

Figure 1.3.   Early fMRI images from Kwong et al. (1992). The left panel shows a set of images starting with the baseline image (top left), and followed by subtraction images taken at different points during either visual stimulation or rest. The right panel shows the timecourse of a region of interest in visual cortex, showing signal increases that occur during periods of visual stimulation.

were evident even from inspection of single subtraction images. In order to obtain statistical evidence for this effect, the images acquired during the stimulation blocks were compared to the images from the no-stimulation blocks using a simple paired t-test. This approach provided an easy way to find activation, but its limitations quickly became evident. First, it required long blocks of stimulation (similar to PET scans) in order to allow the signal to reach a steady state. Although feasible, this approach in essence wasted the increased temporal resolution available from fMRI data. Second, the simple t-test approach did not take into account the complex temporal structure of fMRI data, which violated the assumptions of the statistics.

Researchers soon realized that the greater temporal resolution of fMRI relative to PET permitted the use of event-related (ER) designs, where the individual impact of relatively brief individual stimuli could be assessed. The first such studies used trials that were spaced very widely in time (in order to allow the hemodynamic response to return to baseline) and averaged the responses across a time window centered around each trial (Buckner et al., 1996). However, the limitations of such slow event-related designs were quickly evident; in particular, it required a great amount of scan time to collect relatively few trials. The modeling of trials that occurred more rapidly in time required a more fundamental understanding of the BOLD hemodynamic response (HRF). A set of foundational studies (Boynton et al., 1996; Vazquez & Noll, 1998; Dale & Buckner, 1997) established the range of event-related fMRI designs for which the BOLD response behaved as a linear time invariant system, which was roughly for events separated by at least 2 seconds. The linearity of the BOLD is a crucial result, dramatically simplifying the analysis by allowing the use of the General Linear Model and also allowing the study of the statistical efficiency of various fMRI designs. For example, using linearity Dale (1999) and Josephs & Henson (1999) demonstrated that block designs were optimally sensitive to differences between conditions, but careful arrangement of the events could provide the best possible ER design.

The noise in BOLD data also was a challenge, particularly with regard to the extreme low frequency variation referred to as "drift." Early work systematically examined the sources and nature of this noise and characterized it as a combination of physiological effects and scanner instabilities (Smith et al., 1999; Zarahn et al., 1997; Aguirre et al., 1997), though the sources of drift remain somewhat poorly understood. The drift was modeled by a combination of filters or nuisance regressors, or using temporal autocorrelation models (Woolrich et al., 2001). Similar to PET, global variation in the BOLD signal was observed that was unrelated to the task, and there were debates as to whether global fMRI signal intensity should be regressed out, scaled-away, or ignored (Aguirre et al., 1997).

In PET, little distinction was made between intrasubject and group analyses, and the repeated measures correlation that arises from multiple (at most 12) scans from a subject was ignored. With fMRI, there are hundreds of scans for each individual. An early approach was to simply concatenate the time series for all individuals in a study and perform the analysis across all timepoints, ignoring the fact that these are repeated measures obtained across different individuals. This produced "fixed effects" inferences in which a single subject could drive significant results in a group analysis. The SPM group (Holmes & Friston, 1999) proposed a simple approach to "mixed effects" modeling, whose inferences would generalize to the sampled population. Their approach involved obtaining a separate effect estimate per subject at each voxel and then combining these at a second level to test for effects across subjects. Though still widely in use today, this approach did not account for differences in intrasubject variability. An improved approach was proposed by the FMRIB Software Library (FSL) group (Woolrich et al., 2004b; Beckmann & Smith, 2004) that used both the individual subject effect images and the corresponding standard error images. Although the latter approach provides greater sensitivity when there are dramatic differences in variability between subjects, recent work has shown that these approaches do not differ much in typical single-group analyses (Mumford & Nichols, 2009).

Since 2000, a new approach to fMRI analysis has become increasingly common, which attempts to analyze the information present in patterns of activity rather than the response at individual voxels. Known variously as multi-voxel pattern analysis (MVPA), pattern information analysis, or machine learning, these methods attempt to determine the degree to which different conditions (such as different stimulus classes) can be distinguished on the basis of fMRI activation patterns, and also to understand what kind of information is present in those patterns. A particular innovation of this set of methods is that they focus on making predictions about new data, rather than simply describing the patterns that exist in a particular data set.

1.4 Major components of fMRI analysis

The analysis of fMRI data is made complex by a number of factors. First, the data are liable to a number of artifacts, such as those caused by head movement. Second, there are a number of sources of variability in the data, including variability between individuals and variability across time within individuals. Third, the dimensionality of the data is very large, which causes a number of challenges in comparison to the small datasets that many scientists are accustomed to working with. The major components of fMRI analysis are meant to deal with each of these problems. They include

- **Quality control:** Ensuring that the data are not corrupted by artifacts.
- **Distortion correction:** The correction of spatial distortions that often occur in fMRI images.
- **Motion correction:** The realignment of scans across time to correct for head motion.
- **Slice timing correction:** The correction of differences in timing across different slices in the image.
- **Spatial normalization:** The alignment of data from different individuals into a common spatial framework so that their data can be combined for a group analysis.
- **Spatial smoothing:** The intentional blurring of the data in order to reduce noise.
- **Temporal filtering:** The filtering of the data in time to remove low-frequency noise.
- **Statistical modeling:** The fitting of a statistical model to the data in order to estimate the response to a task or stimulus.
- **Statistical inference:** The estimation of statistical significance of the results, correcting for the large number of statistical tests performed across the brain.
- **Visualization:** Visualization of the results and estimation of effect sizes.

The goal of this book is to outline the procedures involved in each of these steps.

1.5 Software packages for fMRI analysis

In the early days of fMRI, nearly every lab had its own home-grown software package for data analysis, and there was little consistency between the procedures across different labs. As fMRI matured, several of these in-house software packages began to be distributed to other laboatories, and over time several of them came to be distributed as full-fledged analysis suites, able to perform all aspects of analysis of an fMRI study.

Table 1.1.   An overview of major fMRI software packages

Package	Developer	Platforms[a]	Licensing
SPM	University College London	MATLAB	Open-source
FSL	Oxford University	UNIX	Open source
AFNI	NIMH	UNIX	Open source
Brain Voyager	Brain Innovation	Mac OS X, Windows, Linux	Commercial (closed-source)

[a]Those platform listed as UNIX are available for Linux, Mac OS X, and other UNIX flavors.

Today, there are a number of comprehensive software packages for fMRI data analysis, each of which has a loyal following. (See Table 1.1) The Web sites for all of these packages are linked from the book Web site.

1.5.1 SPM

SPM (which stands for Statistical Parametric Mapping) was the first widely used and openly distributed software package for fMRI analysis. Developed by Karl Friston and colleagues in the lab then known as the Functional Imaging Lab (or FIL) at University College London, it started in the early 1990s as a program for analysis of PET data and was then adapted in the mid-1990s for analysis of fMRI data. It remains the most popular software package for fMRI analysis. SPM is built in MATLAB, which makes it accessible on a very broad range of computer platforms. In addition, MATLAB code is relatively readable, which makes it easy to look at the code and see exactly what is being done by the programs. Even if one does not use SPM as a primary analysis package, many of the MATLAB functions in the SPM package are useful for processing data, reading and writing data files, and other functions. SPM is also extensible through its toolbox functionality, and a large number of extensions are available via the SPM Web site. One unique feature of SPM is its connectivity modeling tools, including psychophysiological interaction (Section 8.2.4) and dynamic causal modeling (Section 8.3.4). The visualization tools available with SPM are relatively limited, and many users take advantage of other packages for visualization.

1.5.2 FSL

FSL (which stands for FMRIB Software Library) was created by Stephen Smith and colleagues at Oxford University, and first released in 2000. FSL has gained substantial popularity in recent years, due to its implementation of a number of cutting-edge techniques. First, FSL has been at the forefront of statistical modeling for fMRI data, developing and implementing a number of novel modeling, estimation, and inference techniques that are implemented in their FEAT, FLAME, and RANDOMISE modules. Second, FSL includes a robust toolbox for independent components analysis (ICA; see Section 8.2.5.2), which has become very popular both for artifact detection and for modeling of resting-state fMRI data. Third, FSL includes a sophisticated set of tools for analysis of diffusion tensor imaging data, which is used to analyze the structure of white matter. FSL includes an increasingly powerful visualization tool called FSLView, which includes the ability to overlay a number of probabilistic atlases and to view time series as a movie. Another major advantage of FSL is its integration with grid computing, which allows for the use of computing clusters to greatly speed the analysis of very large datasets.

1.5.3 AFNI

AFNI (which stands for Analysis of Functional NeuroImages) was created by Robert Cox and his colleagues, first at the Medical College of Wisconsin and then at the National Institutes of Mental Health. AFNI was developed during the very early days of fMRI and has retained a loyal following. Its primary strength is in its very powerful and flexible visualization abilities, including the ability to integrate visualization of volumes and cortical surfaces using the SUMA toolbox. AFNI's statistical modeling and inference tools have historically been less sophisticated than those available in SPM and FSL. However, recent work has integrated AFNI with the R statistical package, which allows use of more sophisticated modeling techniques available within R.

1.5.4 Other important software packages

BrainVoyager. Brain Voyager, produced by Rainer Goebel and colleagues at Brain Innovation, is the major commercial software package for fMRI analysis. It is available for all major computing platforms and is particularly known for its ease of use and refined user interface.

FreeSurfer. FreeSurfer is a package for anatomical MRI analysis developed by Bruce Fischl and colleagues at the Massachusetts General Hospital. Even though it is not an fMRI analysis package per se, it has become increasingly useful for fMRI analysis because it provides the means to automatically generate both cortical surface models and anatomical parcellations with a minimum of human input. These models can then be used to align data across subjects using surface-based approaches, which may in some cases be more accurate than the more standard volume-based methods for intersubject alignment (see Chapter 4). It is possible to import statistical results obtained using FSL or SPM and project them onto the reconstructed cortical surface, allowing surface-based group statistical analysis.

1.6 Choosing a software package

Given the variety of software packages available for fMRI analysis, how can one choose among them? One way is to listen to the authors of this book, who have each used a number of packages and eventually have chosen FSL as their primary analysis package, although we each use other packages regularly as well. However, there are other reasons that one might want to choose one package over the others. First, what package do other experienced researchers at your institution use? Although mailing lists can be helpful, there is no substitute for local expertise when one is learning a new analysis package. Second, what particular aspects of analysis are most important to you? For example, if you are intent on using dynamic causal modeling, then SPM is the logical choice. If you are interested in using ICA, then FSL is a more appropriate choice. Finally, it depends upon your computing platform. If you are a dedicated Microsoft Windows user, then SPM is a good choice (though it is always possible to install Linux on the same machine, which opens up many more possibilities). If you have access to a large cluster, then you should consider FSL, given its built-in support for grid computing.

It is certainly possible to mix and match analysis tools for different portions of the processing stream. This has been made increasingly easy by the broad adoption of the NIfTI file format by most of the major software packages (see Appendix C for more on this). However, in general it makes sense to stick largely with a single package, if only because it reduces the amount of emails one has to read from the different software mailing lists!

1.7 Overview of processing streams

We refer to the sequence of operations performed in course of fMRI analysis as a *processing stream*. Figure 1.4 provides a flowchart depicting some common processing streams. The canonical processing streams differ somewhat between different software packages; for example, in SPM spatial normalization is usually applied prior to statistical analysis, whereas in FSL it is applied to the results from the statistical analysis. However, the major pieces are the same across most packages.

1.8 Prerequisites for fMRI analysis

Research into the development of expertise suggests that it takes about ten years to become expert in any field (Ericsson et al., 1993), and fMRI analysis is no different, particularly because it requires a very broad range of knowledge and skills. However, the new researcher has to start somewhere. Here, we outline the basic areas of knowledge that we think are essential to becoming an expert at fMRI analysis, roughly in order of importance.

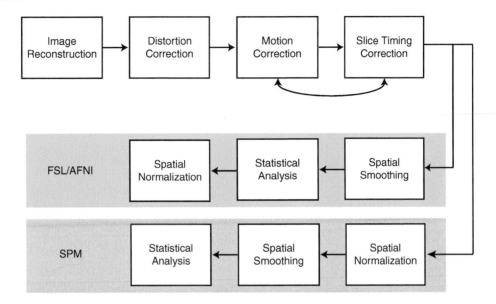

Figure 1.4.   A depiction of common processing streams for fMRI data analysis.

1. *Probability and statistics.* There is probably no more important foundation for fMRI analysis than a solid background in basic probability and statistics. Without this, nearly all of the concepts that are central to fMRI analysis will be foreign.

2. *Computer programming.* It is our opinion that one simply cannot become an effective user of fMRI analysis without strong computer programming skills. There are many languages that are useful for fMRI analysis, including MATLAB, Python, and UNIX shell scripting. The particular language is less important than an underlying understanding of the methods of programming, and this is a place where practice really does make perfect, particularly with regard to debugging programs when things go wrong.

3. *Linear algebra.* The importance of linear algebra extends across many different aspects of fMRI analysis, from statistics (where the general linear model is most profitably defined in terms of linear algebra) to image processing (where many operations on images are performed using linear algebra). A deep understanding of fMRI analysis requires basic knowledge of linear algebra.

4. *Magnetic resonance imaging.* One can certainly analyze fMRI data without knowing the details of MRI acquisition, but a full understanding of fMRI data requires that one understand where the data come from and what they are actually measuring. This is particularly true when it comes to understanding the various ways in which MRI artifacts may affect data analysis.

5. *Neurophysiology and biophysics.* fMRI signals are interesting because they are an indirect measure of the activity of individual neurons. Understanding how

neurons code information, and how these signals are reflected in blood flow, is crucial to interpreting the results that are obtained from fMRI analysis.

6. *Signal and image processing.* A basic understanding of signal and image processing methods is important for many of the techniques discussed in this book. In particular, an understanding of Fourier analysis (Section 2.4) is very useful for nearly every aspect of fMRI analysis.

Image processing basics

Many of the operations that are performed on fMRI data involve transforming images. In this chapter, we provide an overview of the basic image processing operations that are important for many different aspects of fMRI data analysis.

2.1 What is an image?

At its most basic, a digital image is a matrix of numbers that correspond to spatial locations. When we view an image, we do so by representing the numbers in the image in terms of gray values (as is common for anatomical MRI images such as in Figure 2.1) or color values (as is common for statistical parametric maps). We generally refer to each element in the image as a "voxel," which is the three-dimensional analog to a pixel. When we "process" an image, we are generally performing some kind of mathematical operation on the matrix. For example, an operation that makes the image brighter (i.e., whiter) corresponds to increasing the values in the matrix.

In a computer, images are represented as *binary* data, which means that the representation takes the form of ones and zeros, rather than being represented in a more familiar form such as numbers in plain text or in a spreadsheet. Larger numbers are represented by combining these ones and zeros; a more detailed description of this process is presented in Box 2.1.

Numeric formats. The most important implication of numeric representation is that information can be lost if the representation is not appropriate. For example, imagine that we take a raw MRI image that has integer values that range between 1,000 and 10,000, and we divide each voxel value by 100, resulting in a new image with values ranging between 10 and 100. If the resulting image is stored using floating point values, then all of the original information will be retained; that is, if there were 9,000 unique values in the original image, there will also be 9,000 unique

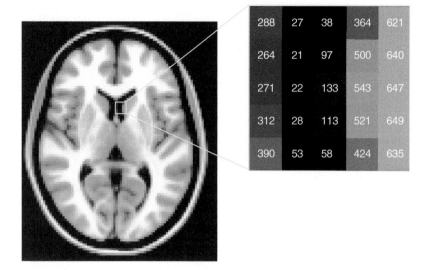

Figure 2.1.   An image as a graphical representation of a matrix. The gray scale values in the image at left correspond to numbers, which is shown for a set of particular voxels in the closeup section on the right.

values in the new image (3,280 becomes 32.8, and so on). If the resulting image is stored instead as integers (like the original image), then information is lost: The 9,000 unique values between 1,000 and 10,000 will be replaced by only 90 unique values in the new image, which means that information has been lost when values are rounded to the nearest integer. The tradeoff for using floating point numbers is that they will result in larger image files (see Box 2.1).

Metadata.   Beyond the values of each voxel, it is also critical to store other information about the image, known generally as *metadata*. These data are generally stored in a *header*, which can either be a separate file or a part of the image file. There are a number of different types of formats that store this information, such as Analyze, NIfTI, and DICOM. The details of these file formats are important but tangential to our main discussion; the interested reader is directed to Appendix C.

 Storing time series data.   Whereas structural MRI images generally comprise a single three-dimensional image, fMRI data are represented as a time series of three-dimensional images. For example, we might collect an image every 2 seconds for a total of 6 minutes, resulting in a time series of 180 three-dimensional images. Some file formats allow representation of four-dimensional datasets, in which case this entire time series could be saved in a single data file, with time as the fourth dimension. Other formats require that the time series be stored as a series of separate three-dimensional datafiles.

Box 2.1 Digital image representation

The numbers that comprise an image are generally represented as either integer or floating point variables. In a digital computer, numbers are described in terms of the amount of information that they contain in *bits*. A bit is the smallest possible amount of information, corresponding to a binary (true/false or 1/0) value. The number of bits determines how many different possible values a numerical variable can take. A one-bit variable can take two possible values (1/0), a two-bit variable can take four possible values ($00, 01, 10, 11$), and so on; more generally, a variable with n bits can take 2^n different values. Raw MRI images are most commonly stored as *unsigned* 16-bit values, meaning that they can take integer values from 0 to 65535 ($2^{16} - 1$). The results of analyses, such as statistical maps, are generally stored as *floating point* numbers with either 32 bits (up to seven decimal points, known as "single precision") or 64 bits up to (14 decimal points, known as "double precision"). They are referred to as "floating point" because the decimal point can move around, allowing a much larger range of numbers to be represented compared to the use of a fixed number of decimal points.

The number of bits used to store an image determines the precision with which the information is represented. Sometimes the data are limited in their precision due to the process that generates them, as is the case with raw MRI data; in this case, using a variable with more precision would simply use more memory than necessary without affecting the results. However, once we apply processing operations to the data, then we may want additional precision to avoid errors that occur when values are rounded to the nearest possible value (known as *quantization* errors). The tradeoff for this added precision is greater storage requirements. For example, a standard MRI image (with dimensions of $64 \times 64 \times 32$ voxels) requires 256 kilobytes of diskspace when stored as a 16-bit integer, but 1,024 kilobytes (one megabyte) when stored as a 64-bit floating point value.

2.2 Coordinate systems

Since MRI images are related to physical objects, we require some way to relate the data points in the image to spatial locations in the physical object. We do this using a *coordinate system*, which is a way of specifying the spatial characteristics of an image. The data matrix for a single brain image is usually three-dimensional, such that each dimension in the matrix corresponds to a dimension in space. By convention, these dimensions (or *axes*) are called X, Y, and Z. In the standard space used for neuroimaging data (discussed further in Section 4.3), X represents the left–right dimension, Y represents the anterior–posterior dimension, and Z represents the inferior–superior dimension (see Figure 2.2).

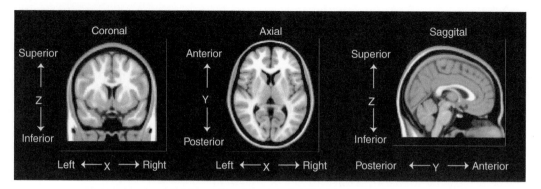

Figure 2.2.   A depiction of the three main axes used in the standard coordinate space for MRI; images taken directly from an MRI scanner may have different axis orientations.

In the data matrix, a specific voxel can be indexed as $[X_{vox}, Y_{vox}, Z_{vox}]$, where these three coordinates specify its position along each dimension in the matrix (starting either at zero or one, depending upon the convention of the particular software system). The specifics about how these data are stored (e.g., whether the first X value refers to the leftmost or rightmost voxel) are generally stored in the image header; see Appendix C for more information on image metadata.

2.2.1 Radiological and neurological conventions

Fields of scientific research often have their own conventions for presentation of data, which usually have arisen by accident or fiat; for example, in electrophysiological research, event-related potentials are often plotted with negative values going upward and positive values going downward. The storage and display of brain images also has a set of inconsistent conventions, which grew out of historical differences in the preferences of radiologists and neurologists. Radiologists prefer to view images with the right side of the brain on the left side of the image, supposedly so that the orientation of the structures in the film matches the body when viewed from the foot of the bed. The presentation of images with the left–right dimension reversed is thus known as "radiological convention." The convention amongst neurologists, on the other hand, is to view images without flipping the left–right dimension (i.e., the left side of the brain is on the left side of the image); this is known as neurological convention. Unfortunately, there is no consistent convention for the storage or display of images in brain imaging, meaning that one always has to worry about whether the X dimension of the data is properly interpreted. Because of the left–right symmetry of the human brain, there are no foolproof ways to determine from an image of the brain which side is left and which is right. Anatomical differences between the two hemispheres are subtle and inconsistent across individuals and do not provide a sufficient means to identify the left and right hemispheres from an image. For the anterior–posterior and inferior–superior dimensions, no convention is needed because it is obvious which direction is up/down or forward/backward due to the anatomy.

2.2.2 Standard coordinate spaces

The coordinate systems discussed earlier provide a link between the physical structures in the brain and the coordinates in the image. We call the original coordinate system in the images as they were acquired from the MRI scanner the *native space* of the image. Although the native space allows us to relate image coordinates to physical structures, the brains of different individuals (or the same individual scanned on different occasions) will not necessarily line up in native space. Different people have brains that are different sizes, and even when the same person is scanned multiple times, the brain will be in different places in the image depending upon exactly where the head was positioned in the scanner. Because many research questions in neuroimaging require us to combine data across individuals, we need a common space in which different individuals can be aligned. The first impetus for such a common space came from neurosurgeons, who desired a standardized space in which to perform stereotactic neurosurgery. Such spaces are now referred to generically as *standard spaces* or *stereotactic spaces*. The most famous of these is the approach developed by Jean Talairach (Talairach, 1967). More recently, a stereotactic coordinate space developed at the Montreal Neurological Institute (MNI) on the basis of a large number of MRI images has become a standard in the field. We discuss these issues in much greater depth in Chapter 4.

2.3 Spatial transformations

Several aspects of fMRI analysis require spatially transforming images in some way, for example, to align images within individuals (perhaps to correct for head motion) or across individuals (in order to allow group analysis).

There is an unlimited number of ways to transform an image. A simple transformation (with a small number of parameters) might move a structure in space without changing its shape, whereas a more complex transformation might match the shape of two complex structures to one another. In general, we will focus on methods that have relatively few parameters in relation to the number of voxels. We will also limit our focus to automated methods that do not require any manual delineation of anatomical landmarks, since these are by far the most common today. In this section, we only discuss *volume-based* transformations, which involve changes to a three-dimensional volume of data. In Chapter 4 on spatial normalization, we will also discuss *surface-based* registration, which spatially transforms the data using surfaces (such as the surface of the cortex) rather than volumes.

Two steps are necessary to align one image to another. First, we have to estimate the transformation parameters that result in the best alignment. This requires that we have a *transformation model* that specifies the ways in which the image can be changed in order to realign it. Each parameter in such a model describes a change to be made to the image. A very simple model may have only a few parameters; such a model will only be able to make gross changes and will not be able to align the fine details of the two images. A complex model may have many more parameters and will be able to align the images better, especially in their finer details. We also need a way to determine how misaligned the two images are, which we refer to as a *cost function*. It is this cost function that we want to minimize in order to find the parameters that best align the two images (see Section 2.3.2).

Once we have determined the parameters of the transformation model, we must then *resample* the original image in order to create the realigned version. The original coordinates of each voxel are transformed into the new space, and the new image is created based on those transformed coordinates. Since the transformed coordinates will generally not fall exactly on top of coordinates from the original image, it is necessary to compute what the intensity values would be at those intermediate points, which is known as *interpolation*. Methods of interpolation range from simple (such as choosing the nearest original voxel) to complex weighted averages across the entire image.

2.3.1 Transformation models

2.3.1.1 Affine transformations

The simplest transformation model used in fMRI involves the use of linear operators, also known as *affine* transformations. A feature of affine transformations is that any set of points that fell on a line prior to the transform will continue to fall on a line after the transform. Thus, it is not possible to make radical changes to the shape of an object (such as bending) using affine transforms.

An affine transformation involves a combination of linear transforms:

- Translation (shifting) along each axis
- Rotation around each axis
- Scaling (stretching) along each axis
- Shearing along each axis

Figure 2.3 shows examples of each of these transformations. For a three-dimensional image, each of these operations can be performed for each dimension, and that operation for each dimension is represented by a single parameter. Thus, a full affine transformation where the image is translated, rotated, skewed, and stretched along each axis in three dimensions is described by 12 parameters.

There are some cases where you might want to transform an image using only a subset of the possible linear transformations, which corresponds to an affine transformation with fewer than 12 parameters. For example, in motion correction we assume that the head is moving over time without changing its size or shape. We can realign these images using an affine transform with only six parameters (three translations and three rotations), which is also referred to as a *rigid*

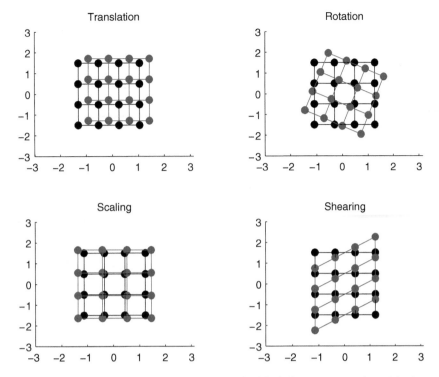

Figure 2.3.   Examples of linear transforms. In each figure, the black dots represent the original coordinate locations, and the blue points represent the new locations after the transformation is applied.

body transformation because it does not change the size or shape of the objects in the image.

2.3.1.2 Piecewise linear transformation

One extension of affine transformations is to break the entire image into several sections and allow different linear transforms within each of those sections. This is known as a *piecewise linear* transformation. Piecewise linear transformations were employed in one of the early methods for spatial normalization of brain images, developed by Jean Talairach (which will be discussed in more detail in Chapter 4).

2.3.1.3 Nonlinear transformations

Nonlinear transformations offer much greater flexibility in the registration of images than affine transformations, such that different images can be matched much more accurately. There is a very wide range of nonlinear transformation techniques available, and we can only scratch the surface here; for more details, see Ashburner & Friston (2007) and Holden (2008). Whereas affine transformations are limited to linear operations on the voxel coordinates, nonlinear transformations allow any kind of operation. Nonlinear transforms are often described in terms of *basis functions*, which are functions that are used to transform the original coordinates. The

---

Box 2.3.1 Mathematics of affine transformations

Affine transformations involve linear changes to the coordinates of an image, which can be represented as:

$$C_{\text{transformed}} = T * C_{\text{orig}}$$

where $C_{\text{transformed}}$ are the transformed coordinates, C_{orig} are the original coordinates, and T is the transformation matrix. For more convenient application of matrix operations, the coordinates are often represented as *homogenous coordinates*, in which the N-dimensional coordinates are embedded in a $(N+1)$-dimensional vector. This is a mathematical trick that makes it easier to perform the operations (by allowing us to write $C_{\text{transformed}} = T * C_{\text{orig}}$ rather than $C_{\text{transformed}} = T * C_{\text{orig}} + \textbf{Translation}$). For simplicity, here we present an example of the transformation matrices that accomplish these transformations for two-dimensional coordinates:

$$C = \begin{bmatrix} C_X \\ C_Y \\ 1 \end{bmatrix}$$

where C_X and C_Y are the coordinates in the X and Y dimensions, respectively. Given these coordinates, then each of the transformations can be defined as follows:

Translation along X ($Trans_X$) and Y ($Trans_Y$) axes:

$$T = \begin{bmatrix} 1 & 0 & Trans_X \\ 0 & 1 & Trans_Y \\ 0 & 0 & 1 \end{bmatrix}$$

Rotation in plane (by angle θ):

$$T = \begin{bmatrix} \cos(\theta) & -\sin(\theta) & 0 \\ \sin(\theta) & \cos(\theta) & 0 \\ 0 & 0 & 1 \end{bmatrix}$$

Scaling along X ($Scale_X$) and Y ($Scale_Y$) axes:

$$T = \begin{bmatrix} Scale_X & 0 & 0 \\ 0 & Scale_Y & 0 \\ 0 & 0 & 1 \end{bmatrix}$$

Shearing along X ($Shear_X$) and Y ($Shear_Y$) axes:

$$T = \begin{bmatrix} 1 & Shear_X & 0 \\ Shear_Y & 1 & 0 \\ 0 & 0 & 1 \end{bmatrix}$$

affine transforms described earlier were one example of basis functions. However, basis function expansion also allows us to re-represent the coordinates in a higher-dimensional form, to allow more complex transformation.

For example, the polynomial basis expansion involves a polynomial function of the original coordinates. A second-order polynomial expansion involves all possible combinations of the original coordinates (X/Y/Z) up to the power of 2:

$$X_t = a_1 + a_2 X + a_3 Y + a_4 Z + a_5 X^2 + a_6 Y^2 + a_7 Z^2 + a_8 XY + a_9 XZ + a_{10} YZ$$

$$Y_t = b_1 + b_2 X + b_3 Y + b_4 Z + b_5 X^2 + b_6 Y^2 + b_7 Z^2 + b_8 XY + b_9 XZ + b_{10} YZ$$

$$Z_t = c_1 + c_2 X + c_3 Y + c_4 Z + c_5 X^2 + c_6 Y^2 + c_7 Z^2 + c_8 XY + c_9 XZ + c_{10} YZ$$

where $X_t/Y_t/Z_t$ are the transformed coordinates. This expansion has a total of 30 parameters ($a_1 \ldots a_{10}$, $b_1 \ldots b_{10}$, and $c_1 \ldots c_{10}$). Expansions to any order are possible, with a rapidly increasing number of parameters as the order increases; for example, a 12th order polynomial has a total of 1,365 parameters in three dimensions.

Another nonlinear basis function set that is commonly encountered in fMRI data analysis is the discrete cosine transform (DCT) basis set, which historically was used in SPM (Ashburner & Friston, 1999), though more recently has been supplanted by spline basis functions. This basis set includes cosine functions that start at low frequencies (which change very slowly over the image) and increase in frequency. It is closely related to the *Fourier transform*, which will be discussed in more detail in Section 2.4. Each of the cosine functions has a parameter associated with it; the lower-frequency components are responsible for more gradual changes, whereas the higher-frequency components are responsible for more localized changes.

For all nonlinear transformations, the greater the number of parameters, the more freedom there is to transform the image. In particular, high-dimensional transformations allow for more localized transformations; whereas linear transforms necessarily affect the entire image in an equivalent manner, nonlinear transforms can change some parts of the image much more drastically than others.

2.3.2 Cost functions

To estimate which parameters of the transformation model can best align two images, we need a way to define the difference between the images, which is referred to as a

T1-weighted MRI   T2-weighted MRI   T2*-weighted fMRI

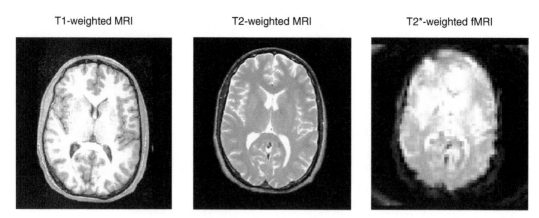

Figure 2.4. Examples of different MRI image types. The relative intensity of different brain areas (e.g., white matter, gray matter, ventricles) differs across the image types, which means that they cannot be aligned simply by matching intensity across images.

cost function. A good cost function should be small when the images are well-aligned and become larger as they become progressively more misaligned. The choice of an appropriate cost function depends critically upon the type of images that you are trying to register. If the images are of the same type (e.g., realigning fMRI data across different timepoints), then the cost function simply needs to determine the similarity of the image intensities across the two images. If the images are perfectly aligned, then the intensity values in the images should be very close to one another (disregarding, for the moment, the fact that they may change due to interesting factors such as activation). This problem is commonly referred to as "within-modality" registration. If, on the other hand, the images have different types of contrast (e.g., a T1-weighted MRI image and a T2-weighted image), then optimal alignment will *not* result in similar values across images. This is referred to as "between-modality" registration. For T1-weighted versus T2-weighted images, white matter will be brighter than gray matter in the T1-weighted image but vice versa in the T2-weighted image (see Figure 2.4), and thus we cannot simply match the intensities across the images. Instead, we want to use a method that is sensitive to the relative intensities of different sets of voxels; for example, we might want to match bright sections of one image to dark sections of another image.

Here we describe several of the most common cost functions used for within- and between-modality registration of MRI images.

2.3.2.1 Least squares

The least-squares cost function is perhaps the most familiar, as it is the basis for most standard statistical methods. This cost function measures the average squared difference between voxel intensities in each image:

$$C = \sum_{v=1}^{n} (A_v - B_v)^2$$

where A_v and B_v refer to the intensity of the vth voxel in images A and B, respectively. Because it measures the similarity of values at each voxel, the least-squares cost function is only appropriate for within-modality registration. Even within modalities, it can perform badly if the two images have different intensity distributions (e.g., one is brighter overall than the other or has a broader range of intensities). One approach, which is an option in the AIR software package, is to first scale the intensity distributions before using the least-squares cost function so that they fall within the same range across images.

2.3.2.2 Normalized correlation

Normalized correlation measures the linear relationship between voxel intensities in the two images. It is defined as

$$C = \frac{\sum_{v=1}^{n}(A_v B_v)}{\sqrt{\sum_{v=1}^{n} A_v^2}\sqrt{\sum_{v=1}^{n} B_v^2}}$$

This measure is appropriate for within-modality registration only. In a comparison of many different cost functions for motion correction, Jenkinson et al. (2002) found that normalized correlation results in more accurate registration than several other cost functions, including least squares. It is the default cost function for motion correction in the FSL software package.

2.3.2.3 Mutual information

Whereas the cost functions described earlier for within-modality registration have their basis in classical statistics, the mutual information cost function (Pluim et al., 2003) (which can be used for between- or within-modality registration) arises from the concept of *entropy* from information theory. Entropy refers to the amount of uncertainty or randomness that is present in a signal:

$$H = \sum_{i=1}^{N} p_i * \log\left(\frac{1}{p_i}\right) = -\sum_{i=1}^{N} p_i * \log(p_i)$$

where p_i is the probability of each possible value x_i of the variable; for continuous variables, the values are grouped into N bins, often called *histogram bins*. Entropy measures the degree to which each of the different possible values of a variable occurs in a signal. If only one signal value can occur (i.e., $p_i = 1$ for only one x_i and $p_i = 0$ for all other x_i), then the entropy is minimized. If every different value occurs equally often (i.e., $p_i = 1/N$ for all x_i), then entropy is maximized. In this way, it bears a

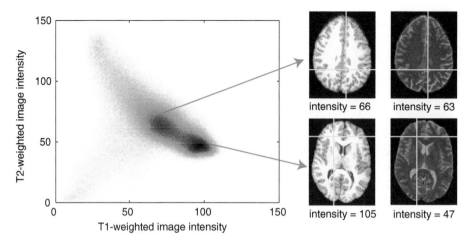

Figure 2.5.   An example of a joint histogram between T1-weighted and T2-weighted images. The darkness of the image indicates greater frequency for that bin of the histogram. The intensities from two different voxels in each image are shown, one in the gray matter (top slices) and one in the white matter (bottom slices).

close relation to the variance of a signal, and also to the uncertainty with which one can predict the next value of the signal. Entropy can be extended to multiple images by examining the *joint histogram* of the images, which plots the frequency of combinations of intensities across all possible values for all voxels in the images (see Figure 2.5). If the two images are identical, then the joint histogram has values along the diagonal only (because the values will be identical in the voxels in each image), whereas differences between the images leads to a greater dispersion of values across the histogram; note that for this within-modality case, correlation would be a more appropriate cost function measure than mutual information (MI). For images from different modalities, where mutual information is more appropriate, greater misregistration leads to greater dispersion in the joint histogram (see Figure 2.6). The *joint entropy* of two images A and B can then be computed from this joint histogram as

$$\mathbf{H(A, B)} = \sum_{i,j} p_{i,j} * \log\left(\frac{1}{p_{i,j}}\right)$$

where i indexes values of A and j indexes values of B, and $p_{i,j} = P(A = A_i \& B = B_j)$. This measure is lowest when the values of an image B are perfectly predictable by the value of the same voxel in image A.

Mutual information is the difference between the total entropy of the individual images and the joint entropy:

$$\mathbf{MI} = H(A) + H(B) - H(A, B)$$

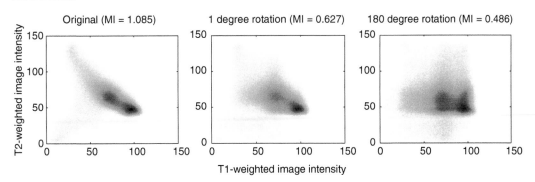

Figure 2.6. Joint histograms for the T1-weighted and T2-weighted images from Figure 2.5. The left panel shows the joint histogram for the original registered images. The middle panel shows the joint histogram after one of the images has been rotated by 1 degree, while the right panel shows the joint histogram after one of the images has been rotated 180 degrees. The MI values for each comparison are presented in the panel labels; MI decreases as the images become less similar.

where $H(A)$ and $H(B)$ are the entropies computed separately for the values in each image respectively (known as *marginal* entropy), and $H(A, B)$ is the joint entropy. Mutual information is greatest when the joint entropy is least, which occurs when the values of one image are maximally predictable from the other image. Thus, mutual information can serve as a measure of similarity between two images.

One potential problem with mutual information is that in some cases, mutual information can increase even as the overlap between images decreases. For this reason, normalization of the mutual information coefficient has been suggested (Studholme et al., 1999):

$$MI = \frac{H(A) + H(B)}{H(A, B)}$$

All of the major software packages (FSL, SPM, and AFNI) offer both regular and normalized mutual information cost functions for image registration.

2.3.2.4 Correlation ratio

The correlation ratio (Roche et al., 1998) measures how well the variance in one measure is captured by the variance in another measure. The correlation ratio for two images A and B is defined as

$$C = \frac{1}{Var(A)} \sum_{k=1}^{N} \frac{n_k}{N} Var(A_k)$$

where k is an index to each unique value of B and N is the number of unique values of B. If the A and B are identical, then across all voxels having some particular value of B there will be no variance in the values of A, and the correlation ratio becomes zero. This measure is similar to the Woods criterion first implemented for PET-MRI coregistration in the AIR software package (Woods et al., 1993), though it does behave differently in some cases (Jenkinson & Smith, 2001). It is suitable for both within-modality and between-modality registration and is the default between-modality cost function in the FSL software package.

2.3.3 Estimating the transformation

To align two images, one must determine which set of parameters for the transformation model will result in the smallest value for the cost function. It is not usually possible to determine the best parameters analytically, so one must instead estimate them using an optimization method. There is an extensive literature on optimization methods, but because fMRI researchers rarely work directly with these methods, we will not describe them in detail here. Interested readers can see Press (2007) for more details. Instead, we will focus on describing the problems that can arise in the context of optimization, which are very important to understanding image registration.

Optimization methods for image registration attempt to find the particular set of parameter values that minimize the cost function for the images being registered. The simplest method would be to exhaustively search all combinations of all possible values for each parameter and choose the combination that minimizes the cost function. Unfortunately, this approach is computationally infeasible for all but the simplest problems with very small numbers of parameters. Instead, we must use a method that attempts to minimize the cost function by searching through the parameter space. A common class of methods perform what is called *gradient descent*, in which the parameters are set to particular starting values, and then the values are modified in the way that best reduces the cost function. These methods are very powerful and can quickly solve optimization problems, but they are susceptible to local minima. This problem becomes particularly evident when there are a large number of parameters; the multidimensional "cost function space" has many local valleys in which the optimization method can get stuck, leading to a suboptimal solution. Within the optimization literature there are many approaches to solving the problem of local minima. Here we discuss two of them that have been used in the neuroimaging literature, regularization, and multiscale optimization.

2.3.3.1 Regularization

Regularization generically refers to methods for estimating parameters where there is a penalty for certain values of the parameters. In the context of spatial normalization, Ashburner, Friston, and colleagues have developed an approach (implemented in SPM) in which there is an increasingly large penalty on more complex warps, using the concept of *bending energy* to quantify the complexity of the warp (Ashburner & Friston, 1999). This means that, the more complex the warp, the more

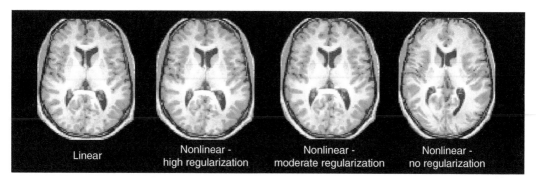

Figure 2.7. An example of the effects of regularization on nonlinear registration. Each of the four images
was created by registering a single high-resolution structural image to the T1-weighted template in SPM5. The leftmost image was created using only affine transformation, whereas
the other three were created using nonlinear registration with varying levels of regularization
(regularization parameters of 100, 1, or 0, respectively). The rightmost panel provides an
example of the kind of anatomically unfeasible warps that result when nonlinear registration
is used without regularization; despite the anatomically infeasible nature of these warps, they
can result in higher-intensity matches to the template.

evidence there needs to be to support it. When using nonlinear registration tools
without regularization (such as AIR and older versions of SPM), it is common to
see radical local warps that are clearly not anatomically reasonable (see Figure 2.7).
The use of regularization prevents such unreasonable warps while still allowing
relatively fine changes that take advantage of small amounts of high-dimensional
warping.

2.3.3.2 Multiscale optimization

The multiscale optimization approach is motivated by the need to search over a
large set of parameter values (to avoid local minima) in a way that is feasible
in a reasonable amount of time. The fundamental idea is to start by estimating
the parameters at relatively low resolution (which will rely on the largest structures in the brain) and then to move to higher resolution once the larger features
have been aligned. For example, in FSL the registration is first performed at a
resolution of 8 mm. Because the rotation parameters turn out to be the most
difficult to estimate, a full search across rotations is performed at this lower
resolution. Once these are determined, then the optimization is performed at
increasingly finer scales (see Figure 2.8), at each step estimating more parameters, until all 12 parameters of the affine transformation are estimated at the
finest level (1 mm). This method was shown to avoid the local minima that can
occur when optimization is performed at a single resolution (Jenkinson & Smith,
2001).

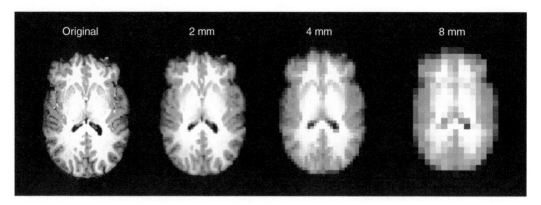

Figure 2.8. An example of the same image sampled at multiple resolutions, as used in multiscale optimization implemented in FSL.

2.3.4 Reslicing and interpolation

Once the parameters for transformation have been estimated, they are then applied to the original image to create a transformed, or *resliced* image. This involves filling in the values of each voxel in the coordinate space using the transformed image coordinates along with the original intensities. If the transformation was limited so that the transformed locations overlapped exactly with locations in the original image, then it would be possible to simply fill in those voxels with the values from the corresponding transformed voxels. However, in general the transformations will involve fractions of voxels; for example, in motion correction the movements being corrected are often less than 1/10 of the voxel's dimensions. In this case, the transformed voxels do not overlap exactly with the original voxels, so it is necessary to interpolate the values of the original image intensities in order to obtain the resliced image.

2.3.4.1 Nearest neighbor interpolation

In nearest neighbor interpolation, the value of the new voxel is replaced with the value of the nearest voxel in the original image. This form of interpolation is rarely used, as it suffers from a number of problems. First, it can result in resliced images that look "blocky" and generally suffer from a loss of resolution. This is especially evident when the interpolation is performed multiple times on the same image, as shown in Figure 2.9. Second, continuous changes in transformation parameters can result in discontinuous changes in cost function values when using nearest neighbor interpolation, which makes it unsuitable for use with optimization methods (which often assume that cost functions are continuous).

The one case in which nearest neighbor interpolation is preferred is to transform images where the voxel values represent labels rather than physical intensities. For example, the anatomical atlases that are included with some software packages are

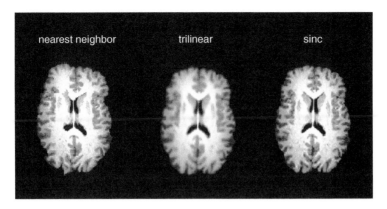

Figure 2.9.   An extreme example of the effects of repeated interpolation. Each image was rotated six times by 0.01 radians, and resliced at each step using nearest neighbor, trilinear, and sinc interpolation, respectively. Note the artifacts in the nearest neighbor image and the increased blurriness in the trilinear image, in comparison to sinc interpolation.

stored as images with specific but arbitrary values corresponding to each structure in the atlas (e.g., voxels in hippocampus have a value of 12, and those in the amygdala have a value of 20). Using an interpolation method that averaged between these numbers would give nonsensical results, so nearest neighbor interpolation would be used to ensure that the label values in the transformed image retain the same exact values as those in the original image.

2.3.4.2 Linear interpolation

This method, often referred to as tri-linear interpolation when it is applied in three dimensions, involves taking a weighted average of the values at each of the nearest points in the original image. An example of linear interpolation is shown in Figure 2.10. This method has the benefit of being relatively fast compared to higher-order interpolation methods, since it only takes into account those points immediately adjacent to the new location. However, it tends to blur the image somewhat more than higher-order interpolation methods, such as sinc interpolation.

2.3.4.3 Higher-order interpolation

A number of interpolation methods have been developed that integrate information across a broader set of voxels than nearest neighbor (which uses only the single nearest voxel) and linear interpolation (which integrates across the eight nearest voxels in three dimensions). The most commonly encountered higher-order interpolation method is *sinc interpolation*, which uses a sinc function [$\mathrm{sinc}(x) = \sin(x)/x$] as shown in FIgure 2.11. In principle this form of interpolation should use information from every voxel in the image, since the sinc function extends to infinity. However,

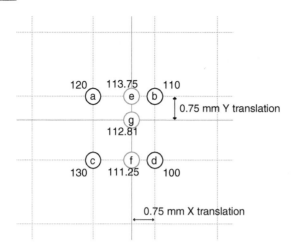

Figure 2.10. An example of linear interpolation. Points a,b, c, and d are the original image locations, on a grid with 2 mm spacing. Point *g* is equivalent to point *b* after a 0.75 mm translation to the left along the *X* dimension and downwards along the *Y* dimension. To determine the intensity of the image at point *g*, one first interpolates along one dimension; in this example, we interpolate along the *X* dimension, finding the values of points *e* and *f*. We then interpolate along the other axis to determine the value at point *g*.

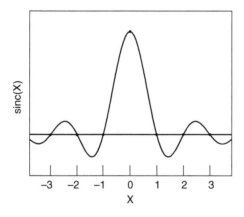

Figure 2.11. An example of the sinc function. The tick marks on the X axis represent the original grid locations, with 0 at the location being interpolated. To obtain the interpolated value, a sinc function (scaled by the image intensity) would be placed at every location on the original grid; the interpolated values are then obtained by adding together all of the sinc function values at the new location. (This is equivalent to convolution of the image by a sinc function.)

this would be computationally very expensive. To make Sinc interpolation is more feasible through the use of a windowed sinc function, wherein the function only extends a limited distance from the point being interpolated, rather than encompass the entire image. There are many different forms of windows that can be applied;

common options include Hanning and rectangular windows. The Hanning window appears to lead to decreased interpolation errors relative to the rectangular window (Ostuni et al., 1997), and thus should be chosen if available, using a window with a radius (or *half-length*) of at least four voxels.

Another form of higher-order interpolation uses basis functions, as we described in Section 2.3.1, for spatial transformation models. Basis functions, such as B-splines, provide a more generalized approach to interpolation, which can encompass nearest-neighbor and linear interpolation as well as higher-order nonlinear interpolation. A detailed description of these methods is beyond the scope of this book; the interested reader is directed to Thevenaz et al. (2000) and Ostuni et al. (1997).

2.4 Filtering and Fourier analysis

Many of the operations that are applied to fMRI data are meant to remove particular kinds of signals or noise from the image. We refer to these operations as *filtering* because they involve the selective transmission of certain kinds of information, just as a coffee filter allows the liquid to pass but retains the solids. Filtering operations are generally specified in the frequency domain rather than the space/time domain, based on the concepts of Fourier analysis.

2.4.1 Fourier analysis

A very general way to understand filtering involves the decomposition of a signal into components. Using Fourier analysis, any signal can be decomposed using a set of periodic functions, such as sines and cosines. An amusing but effective introduction to Fourier analysis can be found in the book *Who Is Fourier?* (Translational College of LEX, 1997), and a more formal introduction can be found in Bracewell (2000). In addition to being important for fMRI data analysis, Fourier analysis also plays a fundamental role in the acquisition of MRI images.

The *Fourier transform* allows one to move from the original signal (in the space or time domain) to a signal in the frequency domain that reflects the strength (or *power*) of component signals at each frequency. When the power is plotted across all frequencies, this is referred to as a *power spectrum*. Power spectra are commonly used in fMRI data analysis. For example, they can be very useful for characterizing the time course of signals that are estimated using independent components analysis (see Chapter 3).

2.4.2 Filtering

Many different types of filters can be applied to data, but most of the filters used in imaging are designed to allow particular portions (or *bands*) of the frequency spectrum to pass through while removing others. *High-pass* filters remove low-frequency information while retaining high-frequency signals, whereas *low-pass* filters do the

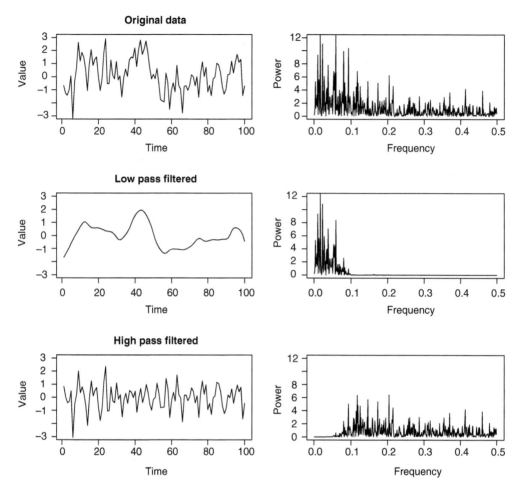

Figure 2.12. An example of Fourier analysis. The plots on the left show a time series, and the plots on the right show the power spectrum for that time series. The top panel shows the original data, the second row shows a low-pass filtered version of the signal, and the third row shows the high-pass filtered version.

opposite. Figure 2.12 shows examples of filtering time series both in the temporal and frequency domains and Figure 2.13 shows examples of the effects of filtering on MRI images.

2.4.3 Convolution

Another way to understand filtering is in terms of the concept of *convolution*. Convolution can be thought of as what happens when a function is passed over another signal and their overlap is added up at each point. For example, we might want to blur an image using a Gaussian function, such that the value at each point in the new image is an average of the surrounding values weighted by the Gaussian. This can be accomplished by convolving the image with a Gaussian function (often referred to as

Original   Low pass   High pass

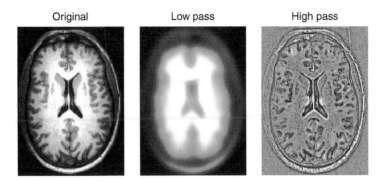

Figure 2.13. Examples of filters applied to a T1-weighted MRI image; the original image is shown at left, and the filtered versions are shown to the right. The low-pass filter blurs the image whereas a high-pass filter enhances the edges in the image.

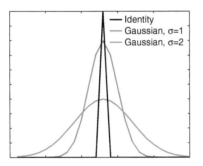 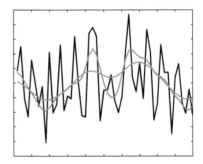

Figure 2.14. An example of convolution. The left panel shows three different kernels used for convolution. The identity kernel has a positive value in its central point and zeros elsewhere, whereas the Gaussian kernels spread gradually from the center. A random signal was created and convolved with each of these kernels, with the results shown in the right panel. Convolution with the identity kernel gives back the original data exactly, whereas convolution with a Gaussian kernel results in smoothing of the data, with greater smoothing for the broader kernel.

a Gaussian *kernel*), as shown in Figure 2.14. The concept of convolution will play a central role in Chapter 5, as it is critical for understanding the relation between neural activity and blood flow in fMRI, where the expected fMRI signal is a convolution between the stimulus function and a hemodynamic response function.

Preprocessing fMRI data

3.1 Introduction

Just as music recorded in a studio requires mixing and editing before being played on the radio, MRI data from the scanner require a number of preprocessing operations in order to prepare the data for analysis. Some of these operations are meant to detect and repair potential artifacts in the data that may be caused either by the MRI scanner itself or by the person being scanned. Others are meant to prepare the data for later processing stages; for example, we may wish to spatially blur the data to help ensure that the assumptions of later statistical operations are not violated. This chapter provides an overview of the preprocessing operations that are applied to fMRI data prior to the analyses discussed in later chapters. The preprocessing of anatomical data will be discussed in Chapter 4.

In many places, the discussion in this chapter assumes basic knowledge of the mechanics of MRI data acquisition. Readers without a background in MRI physics should consult a textbook on MRI imaging techniques, such as Buxton (2002).

3.2 An overview of fMRI preprocessing

Preprocessing of fMRI data varies substantially between different software packages and different laboratories, but there is a standard set of methods to choose from. Figure 3.1 provides an overview of the various operations and the usual order in which they are performed. However, note that none of these preprocessing steps is absolutely necessary in all cases, although we believe that quality control measures are mandatory.

3.3 Quality control techniques

The availability of comprehensive fMRI analysis packages makes it possible to analyze an fMRI data set and obtain results without ever looking closely at the raw data, but

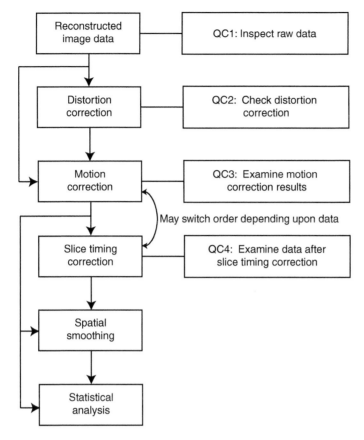

Figure 3.1.   An overview of the standard fMRI preprocessing stream. The appropriate quality control steps are noted at each point. With the exception of motion correction, the rest of the preprocessing steps can be viewed as optional, and their use will depend upon the needs of the study and the available data.

in our opinion it is important for the fMRI researcher to keep a close eye on the raw data and processed data at each step to ensure their quality. Otherwise, one risks falling prey to the old adage: "Garbage in, garbage out." In this section we outline a number of methods that one can use to explore and visualize the presence of artifacts in fMRI data.

3.3.1 Detecting scanner artifacts

A number of artifacts can occur due to problems with the MRI scanner.

Spikes are brief changes in brightness due to electrical instability in the scanner (e.g., due to static electricity discharge). They generally appear as a regular pattern of stripes across the image (see Figure 3.2). Spikes occur relatively infrequently on the current generation of MRI scanners, but when they do occur, they can have large detrimental effects on the analysis.

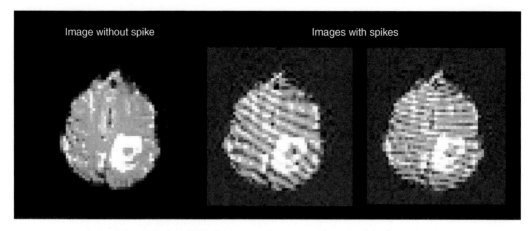

Figure 3.2.   Example of a spike in an fMRI image, reflected by the large diagonal stripes. This image comes from a patient with a brain tumor, which appears as a large white blob at the bottom right side of the brain image. (Images courtesy of Mark Cohen, UCLA)

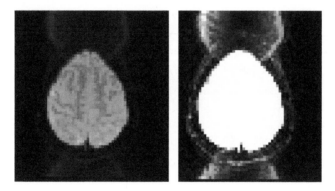

Figure 3.3.   Example of ghosting in an fMRI image. The ghosting is more apparent when the top value in the intensity window of the image viewing program is reduced, as shown in the right panel. (Images courtesy of Mark Cohen, UCLA)

Ghosting occurs when there is a slight offset in phase between different lines of K-space in an echoplanar acquisition and can also occur due to periodic motion such as heartbeat or respiration. It appears as a dim ghost of the brain to each side in the phase-encoded direction of the MRI image (see Figure 3.3). It may be difficult to see ghosting when looking at an image with the brightness window set to the entire range of the image; it can be seen more easily by reducing the top value of the intensity window in the image viewing program (as shown in Figure 3.3). In fMRI, ghosting can result in activation appearing to occur outside of the brain and also cause mislocalization of activation within the brain, if one region of the brain has a ghost in another part. Ghosting rarely causes serious problems for fMRI on the latest generation of MRI systems, but substantial ghosting problems do still occur on occasion. When detected, they should be investigated with your local MRI technician or physicist.

3.3.2 Time series animation

The human eye is very good at detecting changes when an fMRI time series is viewed as an animation. Several tools allow viewing of animated time series; for example, in FSLView, a time series can be viewed as an animation by simply clicking the Movie Mode button. Any glaring changes over time can then be investigated in order to better understand their source; in Chapter 5, we will discuss methods for dealing with bad data points in statistical analysis.

3.3.3 Independent components analysis

As we will see in later chapters, fMRI analysis generally proceeds by creating a statistical model (e.g., a model of task effects) and then finding regions where that model explains the data well. However, sometimes we wish to find signals in the data whose form is unknown, as in the detection of artifacts in fMRI data. There is a set of exploratory data analysis methods that do just this, by detecting systematic patterns in the data; these methods will be described in more detail in Chapter 8 on connectivity modeling, but we introduce them here in the context of artifact detection. These methods decompose the four-dimensional dataset into a set of spatio-temporal components that are mixed together in different proportions to obtain the observed signal. There are many different ways that such a decomposition can be performed, which generally differ in the kinds of constraints that are put upon the components. For example, principal components analysis (PCA) finds a set of components that are orthogonal to one another in multidimensional space, whereas independent components analysis (ICA) finds a set of components that are independent of one another. For a more detailed description of ICA, see Section 8.2.5.2.

ICA has proven very useful for the identification of artifacts in fMRI data. Figure 3.4 shows an example of such an ICA component, detected using the FSL MELODIC ICA tool. ICA is particularly useful for identifying signals related to within-scan effects of head motion or other nonrigid effects of motion, which cannot be removed by standard motion correction techniques.

Once a set of artifactual components is identified, those components can be removed from the data, creating a "denoised" dataset. It is important that such identification of components be based on explicit criteria for rejection to prevent bias; these criteria will generally be based on both the spatial and temporal characteristics of the components. For example, one criterion might be that components will be rejected if they show strong alternation between slices (which is good evidence of a motion-related effect when fMRI data are collected using the common *interleaved* method; see Figure 3.7) along with a timecourse that shows a large spike at one or more timepoints (see Figure 3.4). Methods for the automated classfication of ICA components have been developed which may provide more reliable and unbiased detection of artifact-related components than manual classification (Tohka et al., 2008). However, we have found the manual examination of ICA components to be

Thresholded component map

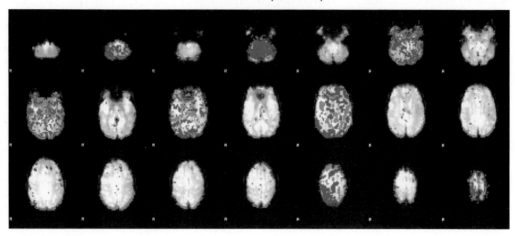

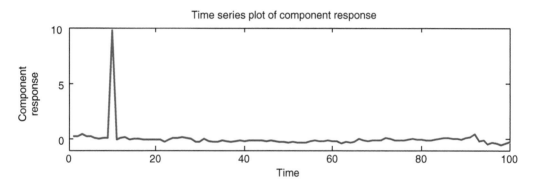

Figure 3.4. An example of a motion-related component detected using FSL's MELODIC ICA tool. The top panels shows a thresholded map that depicts which voxels load significantly on the component, either positively (red) or negatively (blue). Telltale signs of motion include the alternating response between slices (reflecting motion in an interleaved acquisition), coherent positive or negative signals around the edges of the brain, and the presence of a large single spike in the timecourse of the component.

a useful exercise for researchers who are new to fMRI, as it provides a much better view of the variety of signals that may be present in an fMRI dataset.

3.4 Distortion correction

The most common method for fMRI acquisition, gradient-echo echoplanar imaging (EPI), suffers from artifacts near regions where air and tissue meet, such as the sinuses or ear canals. These are due to the inhomogeneity of the main magnetic field (known as *B0*) caused by the air–tissue interfaces, and take two forms: dropout and geometric distortion. Dropout is seen as reduced signal in the brain areas adjacent to these air–tissue interfaces, such as the orbitofrontal cortex and the lateral temporal

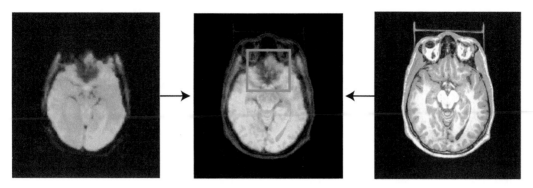

Figure 3.5.   An example of signal dropout in gradient-echo EPI images. The EPI image on the left and the T1-weighted image on the right are combined in the middle (using a transparent overlay in FSLview) to show regions where there is brain tissue in the T1-weighted image but no signal in the EPI image. The orbitofrontal region, which has substantial dropout in this image, is highlighted by the blue box.

lobe (see Figure 3.5). Once the data have been acquired, there is no way to retrieve data from a region with significant dropout, so it is best to employ methods for MRI acquisition that reduce dropout. It is very important to understand the particular dropout patterns that are present in every dataset. For example, one would not want to conclude that the orbitofrontal cortex is not responsive to a particular task manipulation if there is no signal actually present in that region due to dropout. A useful way to appreciate these dropout patterns is to overlay the functional image over a structural image that it has been aligned to (as shown in Figure 3.5).

In addition to signal loss, fMRI images can also be spatially distorted in the same regions. When gradients are applied to encode spatial information in the MRI image, these inhomogeneities in the magnetic field result in errors in the location of structures in the resulting images. Most commonly, regions in the anterior prefrontal cortex and orbitofrontal cortex are distorted. The distortion occurs along the phase encoding direction that is used by the MRI pulse sequence, which is generally the Y (anterior-posterior) axis. These distortions make it difficult to align functional MRI data with structural images.

It is possible to correct somewhat for the effects of magnetic field inhomogeneity using a *field map*, which characterizes the B0 field (Jezzard & Balaban, 1995). Pulse sequences for field mapping are available for most MRI scanners. They generally work by obtaining images at two different echo times. The difference in phase between the two images can be used to compute the local field inhomogeneity, and these values can then be used to create a map quantifying the distance that each voxel has been shifted. By inverting this map, one can determine the original location of the data in each voxel. Figure 3.6 shows an example of distortion correction.

A number of difficulties arise in practice with the use of field maps to unwarp EPI images. First, if there is noise in the field map, then this will introduce noise into

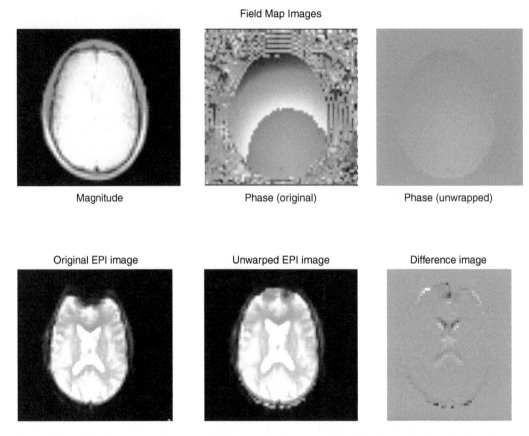

Figure 3.6.   Distortion correction using field mapping. Top panel: Original magnitude and phase images from field mapping scan, along with unwrapped phase map (using FSL's PRELUDE). Bottom panel: Example of original EPI with substantial disortion in the frontal pole, an unwarped version of the same image (using the field map in the top panel), and a difference image obtained by subtracting the unwarped image from the original. (Data from FSL FEEDS dataset)

the unwarped images. One way to address this is to apply some form of low-pass filtering (or *smoothing*) to the field maps, which reduces errors in the unwarped images (Hutton et al., 2002). Second, if the field map is acquired separately from the fMRI time series, then head motion between these scans must be accounted for. It is possible to obtain dual-echo data throughout the fMRI time series, which allows estimation of a unique field map at each timepoint, but this approach is rarely used. There has also been work on methods to combine head motion correction and distortion correction (Andersson et al., 2001), but there are not generally available tools to perform this kind of integrated correction, and it is not clear whether the benefits outweigh the costs of increased complexity.

If distortion correction is employed, then the postcorrection images should be inspected and compared to the precorrection images to ensure that the distortion correction operation has not introduced any artifacts (which can occur if there is a problem with the field map).

3.5 Slice timing correction

Nearly all fMRI data are collected using two-dimensional MRI acquisition, in which the data are acquired one slice at a time. In some cases, the slices are acquired in ascending or descending order. In another method known as *interleaved acquisition* (see Figure 3.7), every other slice is acquired sequentially, such that half of the slices are acquired (e.g., the odd slices) followed by the other half (e.g., the even slices). The use of 2D acquisition means that data in different parts of the image are acquired at systematically different times, with these differences ranging up to several seconds (depending upon the repetition time, or *TR* of the pulse sequence) (see Figure 3.8).

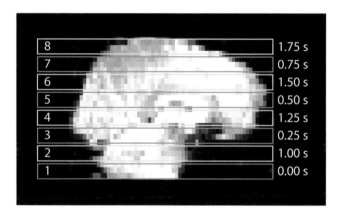

Figure 3.7. A depiction of slice timing in an interleaved MRI acquisition. The slices are acquired in the order 1-3-5-7-2-4-6-8; the times on the right show the relative time at which the data in the slice starts being acquired, assuming a repetition time of 2 seconds.

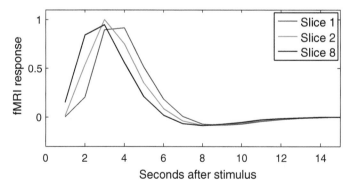

Figure 3.8. The effects of slice timing on the acquired data. The three curves represent samples from the same hemodynamic response at the times corresponding to the slices in Figure 3.7. The slices acquired later in the volume show an apparently earlier response at each time point because the hemodynamic response has already started by the time that they are acquired.

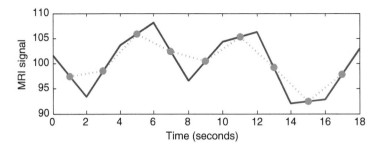

Figure 3.9.   A depiction of slice timing correction. The blue line corresponds to the original time series from a single voxel in the slice acquired at the beginning of each volume acquisition. The red line reflects the interpolated timecourse that would be obtained to correct this slice to match the center slice (which is acquired halfway through the volume, at time $TR/2$). In this example, linear interpolation is used for simplicity; actual slice timing correction methods use sinc interpolation, which will introduce less smoothing in the signal.

These differences in the acquisition time of different voxels are problematic for the analysis of fMRI data. The times of events (such as trials in a task) are used to create a statistical model, which represents the expected signal that would be evoked by the task. This model is then compared to the data at each timepoint; however, this analysis assumes that all data in the image were acquired at the same time, resulting in a mismatch between the model and the data that varies across the brain.

Slice timing correction was developed to address this mismatch between the acquisition timing of different slices (Henson et al., 1999). The most common approach to slice timing correction is to choose a reference slice and then interpolate the data in all other slices to match the timing of the reference slice (see Figure 3.9). This results in a dataset where each slice represents activity at the same point in time. To apply slice timing correction, it is necessary to know the exact timing of the acquistion, which differs across scanners and pulse sequences; this information can generally be obtained from the local physics support personnel.

Despite its seeming appeal, there has been a move away from the use of slice timing correction in practice. One reason is that when it is used, artifacts in one image can be propagated throughout the time series due to the use of sinc interpolation. This is of particular concern in light of the interactions between slice timing and head motion, which will be discussed in more detail in Section 3.6.6. Practical experience also suggests that, with relatively short repetition times ($TR \leq 2$ seconds) and interleaved acquisitions, event-related analysis is relatively robust to slice timing problems. This is particularly likely to be the case when using interleaved acquisition followed by spatial smoothing, since data from adjacent slices (collected 1/2 TR away from one another) are mixed together, resulting in a practical slice timing error of only $TR/2$. Finally, the use of statistical models that include *temporal derivatives*, which allow for some degree of timing misspecification, can also reduce the impact of slice timing differences (see Section 5.1.2).

3.6 Motion correction

Even the best research subjects will move their heads (e.g., due to swallowing), and this motion can have drastic effects on fMRI data, as shown in Figure 3.10. There are two major effects of head motion. First, it results in a mismatch of the location of subsequent images in the time series; this is often referred to as *bulk motion* because it involves a wholesale movement of the head. It is this kind of motion that standard motion correction techniques are designed to correct, by realigning the images in the time series to a single reference image. Bulk motion can have large effects on activation maps, which usually occur at edges in the image; this is due to the fact that large changes in image intensity can occur when a voxel that has no brain tissue in it at one point suddenly contains tissue due to motion. As shown in Figure 3.10, these artifacts can take several forms depending upon the nature of motion, such as a ring of positive or negative activation (reflecting movement along the inferior–superior axis), positive activation on one side of the head and negative activation on the other side (reflecting movement along the left-right axis), or large regions of positive or negative activation in the orbitofrontal cortex (reflecting rotation along the left-right axis). Another common location for such artifacts is at the edges of the ventricles.

Second, head motion can result in disruption of the MRI signal itself. When the head moves, the protons that move into a voxel from a neighboring slice have an excitation that is different from that expected by the scanner, and the reconstructed signal will not accurately reflect the tissue in the voxel; this is known as a *spin history* effect (Friston et al., 1996b). These effects can result in large changes in the intensity of a single slice or set of slices, which can be seen as stripes of alternating bright and dark slices if interleaved acquisition is used. This form of motion cannot be corrected using standard motion correction techniques, but it can potentially

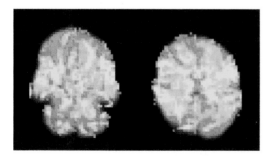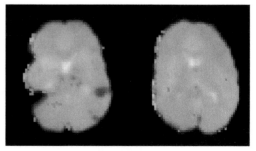

Figure 3.10. Examples of the effects of head motion on the resulting statistical maps. In each case, the image shows activation for a blocked design motor task compared to a resting baseline. The left panel shows a drastic example of motion-related artifacts (from a dataset of an individual with Tourette syndrome). This is often referred to as a "flaming brain" artifact. The right panel shows a more typical example, where motion is seen as activation along one side of the brain, reflecting motion in that direction that is correlated with the task.

be corrected using exploratory methods such as ICA (see Section 8.2.5.2) or using spin-history corrections (Friston et al., 1996b; Muresan et al., 2005).

3.6.1 Stimulus correlated motion

One of the most difficult problems with motion arises when head motion is correlated with the task paradigm, which can occur for a number of different reasons. For example, if the task requires overt speech or movement of large muscle groups, then task-correlated motion should be expected. However, it can also occur in other cases; for example, subjects may become tense during difficult cognitive tasks compared to easy tasks, and this may result in head motion that is correlated with the task. Stimulus-correlated motion is problematic because it can result in changes in activity whose timing is very similar to the timing of the task paradigm, resulting in artifactual activation. Furthermore, because it is so closely correlated with the task, removal of these motion-related signals will often remove task-related signals as well, reducing the sensitivity of the statistical analysis. If the timing of motion is known (as in studies using overt speech), one way to address this issue is to take advantage of the delayed nature of the BOLD response; depending upon the nature of the motion, it may be possible to reduce the correlation between the motion and BOLD response through the use of jittered event-related designs (e.g., Xue et al., 2008).

3.6.2 Motion correction techniques

The goal of motion correction (also known as *realignment*) is to reduce the misalignment between images in an fMRI time series that occurs due to head motion. An overview of the motion correction process is shown in Figure 3.11. In brief, each

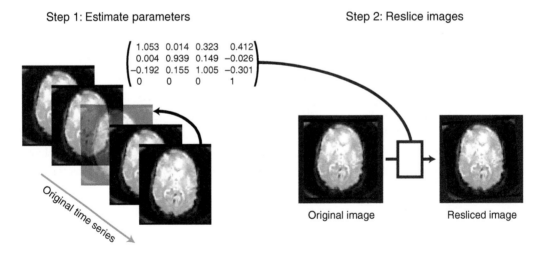

Figure 3.11. An overview of the motion correction process. In the first step, the motion is estimated between each image and the reference, which in this example is the middle image in the time series. In the second step, the parameters obtained for each image are used to create a resliced version of the image that best matches the reference image.

image in the fMRI time series is aligned to a common reference scan using an image registration method, and the images are then resliced in order to create realigned versions of the original data.

Motion correction tools generally assume that head motion can be described using a rigid body transformation, which means that the position of the head can change (by translation or rotation along each of the three axes) but that the shape of the head cannot change. These techniques can thus only correct for bulk motion. However, as noted earlier, when motion occurs during the acquisition of a scan, it can result in disruption of the image intensities, rather than a simple movement of the head in the image. Because these effects cannot be described by rotation or translation of the entire brain, they cannot be corrected by current motion correction methods.

3.6.2.1 Estimating motion

Figure 3.12 shows an example of head motion estimates for an fMRI time series. The plots shown here reflect the parameters of the rigid body transformation that are estimated for each timepoint in comparison to the reference image; note that the parameters are zero at the reference image since it matches itself exactly. Motion correction tools generally provide a plot of these parameters and/or a file that contains the parameters. It can often be useful to transform these estimates to obtain estimates of head displacement from timepoint to timepoint, which is equivalent to the temporal derivative of the motion parameters (see lower panels in Figure 3.12); this can be obtained at each timepoint (from 2 to N) by subtracting the parameter at the previous timepoint.

3.6.2.2 Choosing a target

The target for motion correction can be a specific single image or a mean of the time series. There does not seem to be any appreciable benefit of using a mean image rather than a single image (Jenkinson et al., 2002), and it requires an extra computational step, so it is generally recommended that a single image be used as the reference. When using a single image as a target, it is advisable to use an image from the middle of the time series rather than the first timepoint, for two reasons. First, the middle image should be the closest (on average) to any other image in the time series. Second, the first few images in an fMRI time series sometimes have slightly different contrast (if the magnetization has not yet reached a steady state), which makes them less similar to the rest of the time series.

3.6.2.3 Choosing a cost function

Most motion correction algorithms use a within-modality cost function that is sensitive to the correlation of values between the target and reference images, such as least squares (SPM5) or normalized correlation ratio (FSL 4); see Section 2.3.2 for background on cost functions for image registration. However, when large amounts of activation are present, it is possible that this task-related signal could

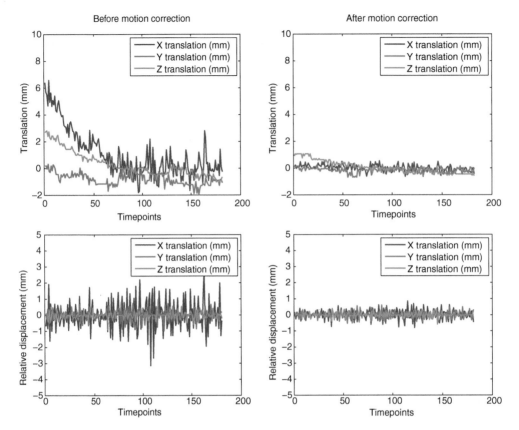

Figure 3.12. Plots of estimated head motion. The top panels plot translation between timepoints, before and after motion correction (i.e., how far the brain is from the reference image). The bottom panels plot the first derivative of the data in the top panels, which correspond to relative displacement at each timepoint (i.e., how far the brain is from the previous timepoint). Relative displacement is often more useful as a means to inspect for motion than absolute translation.

be misinterpreted as motion when such a cost function is used (Freire & Mangin, 2001), resulting in inaccurate motion estimates and errors in the realigned images. Other cost functions such as mutual information or robust estimators may be less sensitive to these effects (Freire et al., 2002). It is not clear how important these effects are in practice. The simulations presented by Friere and Mangin suggest that these effects do not emerge unless relatively large proportions of the brain are strongly active. This suggests that users with tasks that result in large amounts of activation may wish to use a robust cost function such as mutual information for motion correction to prevent contamination of the motion estimates by activation signals.

3.6.2.4 Creating realigned images

A number of possible interpolation methods can be used to create the realigned time series (see Section 2.3.4 for background on these methods). Linear interpolation is relatively fast, but is known to result in a greater amount of smoothing and error in the interpolated images when compared to higher-order methods (Ostuni et al., 1997). Higher-order methods used for interpolation in motion correction include sinc, spline, and Fourier-based interpolation. The practical differences between these methods appear to be small (Oakes et al., 2005), so choices between these methods will likely be driven by considerations such as processing time and availability within a particular package. If processing time is not a concern, then a higher-order method should be used when available, though it should also be noted that the gains in accuracy obtained using a higher-order interpolation method are likely to be swamped by any spatial smoothing that is applied later in the processing stream.

3.6.3 Prospective motion correction

One relatively new development in fMRI methods is the availability of pulse sequences that modify the location of the data acquisition at every timepoint in order to prospectively correct for head motion. This approach has the benefit of creating a motion-corrected dataset without the need for any interpolation. The use of prospective motion correction could be quite beneficial (Thesen et al., 2000), but it is important for users to consider the robustness of these methods for their particular applications. Since the online methods must use quick and thus relatively simple methods for estimating the location of the slices for the next timepoint, there could potentially be error in the predicted slice location which could, for example, cause loss of data from particular brain regions. Because such errors would be more likely in cases of large within-scan motion, these methods may paradoxically be best suited to populations where the motion is relatively minor.

3.6.4 Quality control for motion correction

As with any processing operation, the results should be checked to make sure that the operation was successful and that no additional artifacts were introduced. One useful way to check the results of motion correction is to view the motion-corrected image as a movie; any visible motion in this movie would suggest that the motion correction operation was not completely successful.

It might be tempting to run motion correction multiple times on the same dataset if there are remaining signs of motion following the first application of motion correction. However, this is strongly discouraged. Since the first pass should remove most effects of motion that are amenable to removal, on subsequent runs the algorithm will be much more sensitive to other signals, such as activation-related signals. In addition, the interpolation errors that are introduced at each step will degrade the data.

3.6.5 Interactions between motion and susceptibility artifacts

Motion correction techniques generally use a rigid-body (six-parameter) spatial transformation model, which assumes that the effects of motion do not change the shape of the brain, just its position and orientation. However, in regions of susceptibility artifact, the effects of motion do not obey a rigid-body model. For example, if the head rotates around the X axis (as in swallowing), the angle of slices through the orbitofrontal cortex will change. Because dropout and distortion in this region depend upon the orientation of the slice with respect to the brain, they will differ due to the change in the effective slice angle through the brain, and this will result in differences in the shape of the brain in the image rather than simply differences in the position and orientation of the brain. These changes can result in artifactual activation (Wu et al., 1997), especially if motion is correlated with the task. For this reason, large regions of activation in the orbitofrontal cortex that are very near regions affected by susceptibility artifact should be interpreted with some caution. These problems also provide further motivation for the use of techniques to reduce susceptibility artifacts at the point of data acquisition.

3.6.6 Interactions between motion correction and slice timing correction

Slice timing correction and motion correction can interact with one another, and the nature of these interactions is determined by the order in which they are performed. If motion correction is performed first, then data that were actually acquired at one point in time may be moved to a different slice, and thus the nominal acquisition time that is specified in the slice timing correction algorithm may not match the actual acquisition timing of those data. In addition, if there is a significant amount of through-plane motion or rotation, then the interpolated voxels following motion correction will include a mixture of data acquired at different points in time, again resulting in potential errors due to slice timing correction.

If slice timing correction is performed first, then there is a potential for motion-related intensity differences (which can be very large) to be propagated across time. In addition, any actual through-plane motion or rotation will result in exactly the same kind of mismatch between nominal and actual timing of data acquisition discussed previously. This problem can be somewhat reduced by using prospective motion correction (see Section 3.6.3), which will reduce effects of motion without the need for interpolation and thus without mixing data collected at different times.

We would generally suggest that, if one insists on using slice timing correction, it is applied after motion correction, since the effects of motion on voxel intensity can potentially be very large. However, as noted in Section 3.5, there are good reasons to avoid slice timing correction altogether if data are acquired using a relatively short *TR* (2 seconds or less).

3.6.7 How much is too much motion?

One of the most often asked questions regarding fMRI data analysis is how much motion is too much, such that scans should be thrown away entirely if they exceed that amount. Unfortunately, there is no easy answer to this question. To a large degree, it depends upon how well the effects of motion are described by the rigid body model: Not all motion is created equal. If the motion is gradual or occurs between scanning runs, then a large amount of displacement can be corrected, whereas if sudden motion occurs during a scan, it is likely that there will be effects on image intensity that cannot be corrected using a rigid-body transformation.

As a general rule of thumb, any translational displacement (i.e., translation between two adjacent timepoints) of more than 1/2 of the voxel dimension should cause great concern about the quality of the data. However, this should not be taken as a hard and fast rule; much smaller amounts of motion can cause serious problems, and sometimes even large amounts of motion can be successfully corrected, especially if motion correction is combined with the ICA denoising approach described earlier. In addition, the impact of motion is likely to vary depending upon how correlated it is with the task or stimulus.

It is our opinion that entire scans should be thrown away only as a very last resort. If the entire scan is riddled with large abrupt movements, then there may be no alternative. However, there are a number of strategies that can be used to address motion effects. First, one can attempt to remove coherent motion signals using exploratory methods such as ICA, as described previously. Second, one can include motion-related parameters in the statistical model (as described in Section 5.1.3). Third, one can exclude some timepoints completely by including explanatory variables in the statistical model for the specific timepoints of interest. We have found that these strategies generally allow most scans to be salvaged (at least in normal subject populations), though there will always be some cases where it is necessary to throw away an entire scanning run or subject. In pathological populations or children, it is expected that a significant proportion of data will be unusable due to excessive motion.

3.6.8 Physiological motion

In addition to motion caused by gross movements of the subject's head, there is also significant motion of the brain caused by physiological pulsations related to heartbeat and breathing. The cardiac cycle is faster than than the repetition time of most fMRI acquisitions, which results in *aliasing* of the cardiac cycle to lower frequencies (see Figure 3.13 for a description of aliasing). In addition to pulsatile motion due to the heartbeat, there may also be changes in the image due to respiration; the changes in the magnetic susceptibility within the chest across the respiratory cycle cause small changes in the magnetic field at the head.

One approach to addressing the problem of physiological motion is to monitor and record the timing of heartbeat and respiration during scanning, and then to retrospectively remove these effects from the data (e.g., Glover et al., 2000). These methods are effective but require the added complication of physiological monitoring during scanning. A second approach is to use *cardiac gating*, in which the timing of acquisition of individual image volumes is determined by the subject's

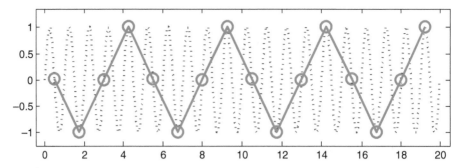

Figure 3.13. Aliasing occurs when a dataset contains periodic signals at frequencies higher than the *Nyquist frequency*, which is half the sampling frequency. For example, if the frequency of heartbeats is once per second, then it would be necessary to sample at least twice per second to prevent aliasing of the heatbeat signal to lower frequencies. In this figure, the 1.0-Hz (once every second) heartbeat signal, shown in blue, is aliased to a lower frequency of 0.2 Hz when sampled at a rate of once every 1.25 seconds (0.8 Hz), shown in red.

own heartbeat. This method has been particularly useful in obtaining images from deep brain structures such as the superior colliculus (Guimaraes et al., 1998), which show the greatest amount of motion due to pulsatility. However, it has a number of limitations (such as a nonstationary *TR*) that make data analysis difficult, and it can also be technically difficult to implement for fMRI scanning. Another more general approach is to use ICA to detect artifactual components in the fMRI time series, as discussed earlier. This method is likely to detect some of the effects of physiological motion, though not as well as methods that use physiological monitoring; however, it has the benefit of not requiring any additional data collection beyond the standard fMRI acquisition.

3.7 Spatial smoothing

Spatial smoothing involves the application of a filter to the image, which removes high-frequency information (see Section 2.4 for background on filtering). It may seem unintuitive that, having put so much effort into acquiring fMRI data with the best possible resolution, we would then blur the images, which amounts to throwing away high-frequency information. However, there are a number of reasons researchers choose to apply spatial smoothing to fMRI data. First, by removing high-frequency information (i.e., small-scale changes in the image), smoothing increases the signal-to-noise ratio for signals with larger spatial scales. Because most activations in fMRI studies extend across many voxels, the benefits of gain in signal for larger features may outweigh the costs of losing smaller features. In addition, the acquisition of smaller voxels can help reduce dropout in regions of susceptibility artifacts, and smoothing can help overcome the increased noise that occurs when small voxels are used. Second, when data are combined across individuals, it is known that there is variability in the spatial location of functional regions that is not corrected by spatial normalization (for more details, see Chapter 4). By blurring the data across space, spatial smoothing can help reduce the mismatch across individuals, at the expense of spatial resolution. Third, there are some analysis methods (in particular, the theory of Gaussian random fields; see Section 7.3.1.2) that require a specific degree of spatial smoothness. Whereas spatial smoothing is almost always applied for standard group fMRI studies, there are some cases in which unsmoothed data are analyzed, such as the pattern classification analyses described in Chapter 9.

The most common means of spatial smoothing is the convolution of the three-dimensional image with a three-dimensional Gaussian filter (or *kernel*); see Section 2.4.3 for more on convolution). The amount of smoothing imposed by a Gaussian kernel is determined by the width of the distribution. In statistics this is generally described in terms of the standard deviation, whereas in image processing the width of the distribution is described by the full width at half-maximum (or *FWHM*). This measures the width of the distribution at the point where it is at half of its maximum; it is related to the standard deviation (σ) by the equation $FWHM = 2\sigma\sqrt{2\ln(2)}$, or approximately $2.55 * \sigma$. The larger *FWHM*, the greater the smoothing, as was shown in Figure 2.14.

Importantly, the *smoothness* of an image is not necessarily identical to the *smoothing* that has been applied to the image. Smoothness describes the correlations between neighboring voxels. An image with random noise will have a very low amount of smoothness, but MRI images generally have a greater amount of smoothness, both due to filtering applied during image reconstruction and due to the presence of intrinsic correlations in the image. When smoothing is applied to an image, the smoothness of the resulting image is

$$FWHM = \sqrt{FWHM^2_{intrinsic} + FWHM^2_{applied}}$$

This is particularly important to keep in mind when using statistical methods that require an estimate of the smoothness of an image, which will be discussed in more detail in Chapter 7.

3.7.1 How much should I smooth?

There is no magic answer to the question of how much smoothing to apply, in part because there are many reasons to smooth and each may suggest a different answer to the question.

- If you are smoothing to reduce noise in the image, then you should apply a filter that is no larger than the activation signals that you want to detect. Figure 3.14 shows the effects of different filter widths on the resulting activation images. Note, however, that the effects here are specific to the particular task and systems being imaged; if the task resulted in activation of smaller structures, then the same filter width that results in detection here might lead the signal to be lost.

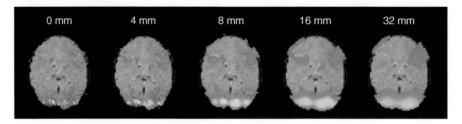

Figure 3.14. An example of the effects of spatial smoothing on activation; the numbers correspond to the FWHM of the smoothing kernel applied to the data before analysis. Increasing smoothing leads to greater detection of larger clusters but decreased detection of smaller clusters.

- If you are smoothing to reduce the effects of anatomical variability, then the optimal smoothing width will depend upon the amount of variability in the population you are imaging, and the degree to which this variability can be reduced by your spatial normalization methods (see Chapter 4 for more on this topic).
- If you are smoothing to ensure the validity of Gaussian random field theory for statistical analysis, then an *FWHM* of twice the voxel dimensions is appropriate.

In general, we would recommend erring toward too little rather than too much smoothing, and we would thus recommend twice the voxel dimensions as a reasonable starting point.

Spatial normalization

4.1 Introduction

In some cases fMRI data are collected from an individual with the goal of understanding that single person; for example, when fMRI is used to plan surgery to remove a tumor. However, in most cases, we wish to generalize across individuals to make claims about brain function that apply to our species more broadly. This requires that data be integrated across individuals; however, individual brains are highly variable in their size and shape, which requires that they first be transformed so that they are aligned with one another. The process of spatially transforming data into a common space for analysis is known as *intersubject registration* or *spatial normalization.*

In this chapter we will assume some familiarity with neuroanatomy; for those without experience in this domain, we discuss a number of useful atlases in Section 10.2. Portions of this chapter were adapted from Devlin & Poldrack (2007).

4.2 Anatomical variability

At a gross level, the human brain shows remarkable consistency in its overall structure across individuals, although it can vary widely in its size and shape. With the exception of those suffering genetic disorders of brain development, every human has a brain that has two hemispheres joined by a corpus callosum whose shape diverges relatively little across individuals. A set of major sulcal landmarks (such as the central sulcus, sylvian fissure, and cingulate sulcus) are present in virtually every individual, as are a very consistent set of deep brain structures such as the basal ganglia. However, a closer look reveals that there is a great deal of variability in the finer details of brain structure. For example, all humans have a transverse gyrus in the superior temporal lobe (known as Heschl's gyrus) that is associated with the primary auditory cortex, but the number and size of these transverse gyri varies considerably across individuals (Penhune et al., 1996; Rademacher et al., 2001). Even in identical twins there can be substantial differences between structures (Toga & Thompson, 2005). The goal of spatial normalization is to transform the brain images from each individual in order to reduce the variability between individuals and allow meaningful group analyses to be successfully performed.

4.3 Coordinate spaces for neuroimaging

To align individuals, we first need a reference frame in which to place the different individuals. The idea of using a three-dimensional Cartesian coordinate space as a common space for different brains was first proposed by the neurosurgeon Jean Talairach (1967). He proposed a "three-dimensional proportional grid" (see Figure 4.1), which is based on a set of anatomical landmarks: The anterior commissure (AC), and posterior commissure (PC), the midline saggital plane, and the exterior boundaries of the brain at each edge.   Given these landmarks, the origin (zero-point) in the three-dimensional space is defined as the point where the AC intersects the midline saggital plane. The axial plane is then defined as the plane along the AC/PC line that is orthogonal to the midline saggital plane, and the coronal plane is defined as the the plane that is orthogonal to the saggital and axial planes. In addition, the space has a *bounding box* that specifies the extent of the space in each dimension, which is defined by the most extreme portions of the brain in each direction (as shown in Figure 4.1).

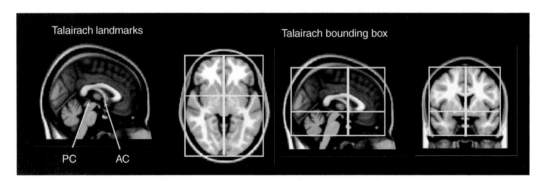

Figure 4.1.   Talairach space is defined by a number of landmarks. The left panel points to the location of the anterior commissure (AC) and posterior commissure (PC), which are the two landmarks that determine the angle of the bounding box around the X axis. The right panel shows the bounding box for the Talairach space, which is determined by the AC and PC, along with the midline saggital plane (which determines the angle around the Z axis) and the superior and inferior boundaries of the cortex (the temporal lobes on the inferior boundary determine the angle around the Y axis).

4.4 Atlases and templates

An *atlas* provides a guide to the location of anatomical features in a coordinate space. A *template* is an image that is representative of the atlas and provides a target to which individual images can be aligned. A template can comprise an image from a single individual or an average of a number of individuals. Whereas atlases are useful for localization of activation and interpretation of results, templates play a central role in the spatial normalization of MRI data. Here we will focus primarily on templates; in Chapter 10, we will discuss atlases in greater detail.

4.4.1 The Talairach atlas

The best-known brain atlas is the one created by Talairach (1967) and subsequently updated by Talairach & Tournoux (1988). This atlas provided a set of saggital, coronal, and axial sections that were labeled by anatomical structure and Brodmann's areas. Talairach also provided a procedure to normalize any brain to the atlas, using the set of anatomical landmarks described previously (see Section 4.7.1 for more on this method). Once data have been normalized according to Talairach's procedure, the atlas provides a seemingly simple way to determine the anatomical location at any particular location.

While it played a seminal role in the development of neuroimaging, the Talairach atlas and the coordinate space associated with it are problematic (Devlin & Poldrack, 2007). In Section 10.2 we discuss the problems with this atlas in greater detail. With regard to spatial normalization, a major problem is that there is no MRI scan available for the individual on whom the atlas is based, so an accurate MRI template cannot be created. This means that normalization to the template requires the identification of anatomical landmarks that are then used to guide the normalization; as we will describe later, such *landmark-based* normalization has generally been rejected in favor of automated registration to image-based templates.

4.4.2 The MNI templates

Within the fMRI literature, the most common templates used for spatial normalization are those developed at the Montreal Neurological Institute, known as the *MNI templates*. These templates were developed to provide an MRI-based template that would allow automated registration rather than landmark-based registration. The first widely used template, known as *MNI305*, was created by first aligning a set of 305 images to the Talairach atlas using landmark-based registration, creating a mean of those images, and then realigning each image to that mean image using a nine-parameter affine registration (Evans et al., 1993). Subsequently, another template, known as ICBM-152, was developed by registering a set of higher-resolution images to the MNI305 template. Versions of the ICBM-152 template are included with each of the major software packages. It is important to note that there are slight differences between the MNI305 and ICBM-152 templates, such that the resulting images may differ in both size and positioning depending upon which template is used (Lancaster et al., 2007).

4.5 Preprocessing of anatomical images

Most methods for spatial normalization require some degree of preprocessing of the anatomical images prior to normalization. These operations include the correction of low-frequency artifacts known as *bias fields*, the removal of non-brain tissues, and the segmentation of the brain into different tissue types such as gray matter, white matter, and cerebrospinal fluid (CSF). The use of these methods varies substantially between software packages.

4.5.1 Bias field correction

Images collected at higher field strengths (3T and above) often show broad variation in their intensity, due to inhomogeneities in the excitation of the head caused by a number of factors (Sled & Pike, 1998). This effect is rarely noticeable in fMRI data (at least those collected at 3T), but can be pronounced in the high-resolution T1-weighted anatomical images that are often collected alongside fMRI data. It is seen as a very broad (low-frequency) variation in intensity across the image, generally brighter at the center and darker toward the edges of the brain. Because this artifact can cause problems with subsequent image processing (such as registration, brain extraction, or tissue segmentation), it is often desirable to correct these nonuniformities.

A number of different methods for bias field correction have been published, which can be broken into two different approaches. The simpler approach is to apply a high-pass filter to remove low-frequency signals from the image (Cohen et al., 2000). A more complex approach combines bias field correction with tissue segmentation; different classes of tissue (gray matter, white matter, and CSF) are modeled, and the algorithm attempts to equate the distributions of intensities in these tissue classes across different parts of the brain (Sled et al., 1998; Shattuck et al., 2001). An example of bias field correction is presented in Figure 4.2. A systematic comparison between these different methods (Arnold et al., 2001) found that the latter approach, which takes into account local information in the image, outperformed methods using global filtering.

4.5.2 Brain extraction

Some (though not all) preprocessing streams include the step of brain extraction (also known as skull-stripping). Removal of the skull and other non-brain tissue can be performed manually, but the procedure is very time consuming. Fortunately, a number of automated methods have been developed to perform brain extraction.

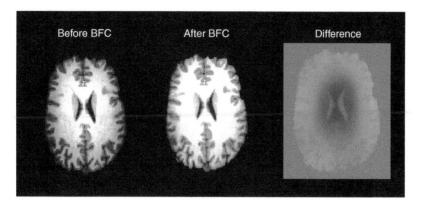

Figure 4.2.   An example of bias field correction. The left panel shows a T1-weighted MRI collected at 3T; the bias field is seen in the fact that white matter near the center of the brain is brighter than white matter toward the edge of the brain. The center panel shows the same image after bias field correction using the BFC software (see the Web site for a current link to this software). The right panel shows the difference between those two images; regions toward the center of the brain have become darker whereas those toward the edges have become brighter.

Some of these (e.g., SPM) obtain the extracted brain as part of a more general tissue segmentation process (as described in the following section), whereas most are developed specifically to determine the boundary between brain and non-brain tissues. It should be noted that the brain extraction problem is of greater importance (and greater difficulty) for anatomical images (where the scalp and other tissues outside the brain have very bright signals) than for functional MRI data (where tissues outside the brain rarely exhibit bright signal).

A published comparison of a number of different brain extraction algorithms (BSE, BET, SPM, and McStrip) suggests that all perform reasonably well on T1-weighed anatomical images, but that there is substantial variability across datasets (Boesen et al., 2004); thus, the fact that an algorithm works well on one dataset does not guarantee that it will work well on another. Most of these algorithms also have parameters that will need to be adjusted to perform well for the particular dataset being processed. It is important to perform quality control checks following the application of brain extraction tools, to ensure that the extraction has worked properly; any errors in brain extraction will likely cause problems with spatial normalization later on.

4.5.3 Tissue segmentation

Another operation that is applied to anatomical images in some preprocessing streams is the segmentation of brain tissue into separate tissue compartments (gray matter, white matter, and CSF). Given the overall difference in the intensity of these different tissues in a T1-weighted MRI image, it might seem that one could simply choose values and threshold the image to identify each component. However, in reality, accurate brain segmentation is one of the more difficult problems in the processing of MRI images. First, MRI images are noisy; thus, even if the mean intensity of voxels in gray matter is very different from the mean intensity of voxels in white matter, the distributions of their values may overlap. Second, there are many voxels that contain a mixture of different tissue types in varying proportion; this is known as a *partial volume effect* and results in voxels with a broad range of intensity depending upon their position. Third, as noted previously there may be nonuniformities across the imaging field of view, such that the intensity of white matter in one region may be closer to that of gray matter in another region than to that of white matter in that other region. All of these factors make it very difficult to determine the tissue class of a voxel based only on its intensity.

There is a very large literature on tissue segmentation with MRI images, which we will not review here; for a review of these methods, see Clarke et al. (1995). One recent approach that is of particular interest to fMRI researchers (given the popularity of the SPM software) is the unified segmentation approach developed by Ashburner & Friston (2005) that is implemented in SPM. This method combines spatial normalization and bias field correction with tissue segmentation, so that the prior probability that any voxel contains gray or white matter can be determined using a probabilistic atlas of tissue types; this prior probability is then combined with the data from the image determine the tissue class. Using this approach, two voxels with identical intensities can be identified as different tissue types (e.g., if one is in a location that is strongly expected to be gray matter and another strong expected to white matter).

4.6 Processing streams for fMRI normalization

There are two commonly used processing streams for spatial normalization of fMRI data (see Figure 4.3); for the purposes of this discussion, we will focus exclusively on template-based normalization methods since they comprise the large majority of current methods. In the first (which is customary in SPM), which we will refer to as *prestatistics normalization*, the data are preprocessed and spatially normalized prior to statistical analysis. In the *poststatistics normalization* approach (used in FSL), the data are preprocessed and the statistical analysis is performed on data in the native space; normalization is applied to the statistical result images following analysis. Each processing stream is valid; choices between them are usually driven by the software package used for analysis. The poststatistics normalization approach is more economical with regard to disk space; since the resolution of the standard space is generally $2\,mm^3$ whereas the resolution of the native space data is generally 3–$4\,mm^3$, it takes substantially more space to store a normalized image versus a native space image. One potential pitfall of the poststatistics approach can arise if there are voxels outside the brain whose values are stored as

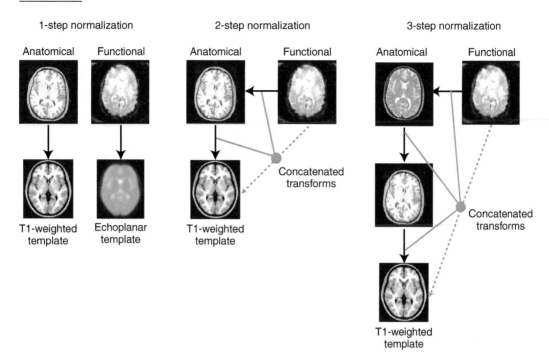

Figure 4.3.   Three common processing streams for spatial normalization of fMRI data. Dark arrows denote direct spatial registration, solid gray arrows represent inclusion of normalization parameters in concatenation, and dotted gray arrow represents implicit normalization obtained by concatenating individual transformation parameters.

NaN ("not a number"), as was the case in older versions of SPM. It is not possible to interpolate over voxels that have NaN values, so any attempt to perform normalization on these images will lead to voxels near the edge of the brain also being set to NaN (since interpolation at the edges will necessarily include voxels outside of the brain). It is possible to solve this problem by replacing the NaN values with zeros in the image, using tools such as SPM's imcalc tool or FSL's fslmaths program.

A second question arises in the choice of which images to use for normalization (see Figure 4.3). The simplest form of registration would be to directly normalize the fMRI data to a template in the appropriate coordinate space made from the same kind of image. This approach is common among users of SPM, which includes an EPI template aligned to the MNI space. However, this approach is not optimal due to the lack of anatomical details in the fMRI images, which means that the registration will be largely driven by the high-contrast features at the edges of the brain. Thus, although the overall outline of the brain will be accurate, structures within the brain may not be accurately aligned.

An alternative is to use a multistep method that utilizes anatomical images in addition to the fMRI images. Most fMRI datasets include, in addition to the fMRI data, a high-resolution anatomical image (which we refer to as a *high-res* image) as well as an anatomical image that covers exactly the same slices as the fMRI acquisition (which we refer to as a *coplanar* image). In the multistep method, the fMRI data are first registered to the subject's anatomical image, which is often referred to as *coregistration*. This is generally performed using an affine transformation with either seven parameters ($X/Y/Z$ translation/rotation and a single global scaling factor) or nine parameters ($X/Y/Z$ translation/rotation/scaling). If both coplanar and high-res images are available, then the best approach is to first align the fMRI data and the coplanar image, then to align the coplanar image to the high-res image, and then to normalize the high-res image to standard space. These transformations (fMRI $\Rightarrow$ coplanar, coplanar $\Rightarrow$ high-res, and high-res $\Rightarrow$ standard space) can then be concatenated to create a single transformation from fMRI native space to standard space (e.g., using the ConcatXFM_gui program in FSL). Creating a single transformation by concatenating transforms, rather than transforming and reslicing the fMRI images at each step, reduces the errors and blurring that accrue with each interpolation. If it is necessary to perform multiple interpolations serially on the same images, then care should be taken to use a higher-order interpolation method such as sinc interpolation to minimize errors and blurring.

4.7 Spatial normalization methods

4.7.1 Landmark-based methods

The first methods developed for spatial normalization used landmarks to align the brains across individuals. The best known such method is the one developed by Talairach, which relied upon a set of anatomical landmarks including the anterior and posterior commisures, midline saggital plane, and the exterior boundaries of the brain in each direction (see Figure 4.1). (In the early days of fMRI, spatial normalization was often referred to generically as "Talairach-ing.") Although landmark-based methods are still available in some software packages (such as AFNI), they have in generally been supplanted by volume-based and surface-based methods.

4.7.2 Volume-based registration

By far the most common form of spatial registration used in fMRI today is volume-based registration to a template image. The methods used for this registration were described in Chapter 2 and include affine linear registration as well as various forms of nonlinear registration. The most common templates are the MNI305 or MNI152, which are averages of large numbers of individuals who have been registered into a common space.

4.7.3 Computational anatomy

A set of approaches from the field known as *computational anatomy* has gained substantial interest due to their ability to effectively align structures across individuals in a way that respects anatomical constraints (Miller, 2004; Toga & Thompson, 2001). Whereas the methods described so far use mathematical basis functions to deform brains to match one another without regard to the nature of the material being warped, computational anatomy methods generally use models based on physical phenomena, such as the deformation of elastic materials or the flow of viscous fluids (Christensen et al., 1994; Holden, 2008). One particular set of approaches use a specific kind of transformation known as a diffeomorphism (for "differentiable homeomorphism"). The mathematics of these methods are quite complex, and we will only provide a brief overview; the interested reader is referred to Miller (2004) and Holden (2008). A diffeomorphic transformation from one image to another can be represented as a *vector field*, where the vector at every point describes the movement of the data in that voxel from the original to the transformed image (see Figure 4.4). These transformations have a very high number of parameters, but they are regularized to ensure that the deformations are smooth and do not violate the topology of the structures being transformed.

Computational anatomy methods have been made widely available via the DARTEL toolbox for SPM (Ashburner, 2007) and the FNIRT tool within FSL. The results from normalization with the DARTEL method are shown in Figure 4.5. Whereas the average of eight individuals after registration using affine or basis-function

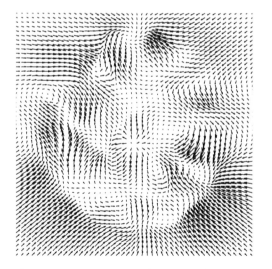
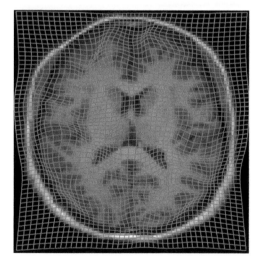

Figure 4.4. An example of the warp field for a brain normalized using FSL's FNIRT nonlinear registration tool. The left panel shows the warp vector field; the arrow at each voxel represents the movement of data in the original image to the transformed image. The right panel shows the normalized image with a warped version of the original image grid overlaid on the image.

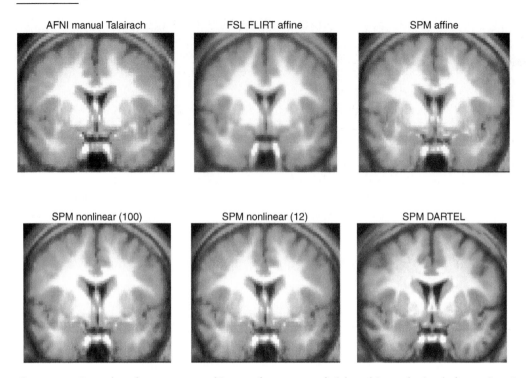

Figure 4.5.   Examples of mean structural images for a group of eight subjects obtained after registration using various registration methods. The number specified for the SPM nonlinear registrations refers to the nonlinear frequency cutoff; a higher number reflects a smaller degree of nonlinear warping. Note, in particular, the relative clarity of the DARTEL image compared to the other images, which reflects the better registration of the different brains using that method.

registration is clearly blurry due to misregistration of fine structure across individuals, the average of these same individuals after registration using DARTEL is much clearer, reflecting better alignment. We expect that these methods will gain greater adoption in the fMRI literature.

4.8 Surface-based methods

Surface-based normalization methods take advantage of the fact that the cerebral cortex is a connected sheet. These methods involve the extraction of the cortical surface and normalization based on surface features, such as sulci and gyri. There are a number of methods that have been proposed, which are implemented in freely available software packages including FreeSurfer and CARET (see book Web site for links to these packages).

The first step in surface-based normalization is the extraction of the cortical surface from the anatomical image (see Figure 4.6). This process has been largely automated in the FreeSurfer software package, though it is generally necessary to ensure that the extracted surface does not contain any topological defects, such as *handles* (when two separate parts of the surface are connected by a tunnel) or *patches*

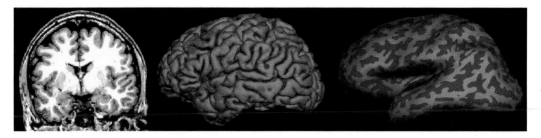

Figure 4.6.   An example of cortical surface extraction using FreeSurfer. The left panel shows the extracted cortical surface in red overlaid on the anatomical image used to extract the surface. The middle panel shows a rendering of the reconstructed surface, and the right panel shows an inflated version of the same surface; light gray areas represent gyri and darker areas represent sulci. (Images courtesy of Akram Bakkour, University of Texas)

(holes in the surface). Once an accurate cortical surface has been extracted, then it can be registered to a surface atlas, and the fMRI data can be mapped into the atlas space after coregistration to the anatomical image that was used to create the surface. Group analysis can then be performed in the space of the surface atlas.

Surface-based registration appears to more accurately register cortical features than low-dimensional volume-based registration (Fischl et al., 1999; Desai et al., 2005), and it is a very good method to use for neuroscience questions that are limited to the cortex. It has the drawback of being limited only to the cortical surface; thus, deep brain regions cannot be analyzed using these methods. However, recent work has developed methods that combine surface and volume-based registration (Postelnicu et al., 2009), and one of these methods is available in the FreeSurfer software package.

Surface-based methods have not been directly compared to high-dimensional volume-based methods such as DARTEL or FNIRT, and those methods may approach the accuracy of the surface-based or hybrid surface/volume-based methods.

4.9 Choosing a spatial normalization method

Given all of this, how should one go about choosing a method for spatial normalization? Because most researchers choose a single software package to rely upon for their analyses, the primary factor is usually availability within the software package that one uses. With the widespread implementation of the NIfTi file format (see Appendix A), it has become easier to use different packages for different parts of the analysis stream, but it still remains difficult in many cases to mix and match different packages. Both SPM and FSL include a set of both linear and nonlinear registration methods; AFNI appears at present to only support affine linear registration. There are also a number of other freely available tools that implement different forms of nonlinear registration. The effects of normalization methods on functional imaging

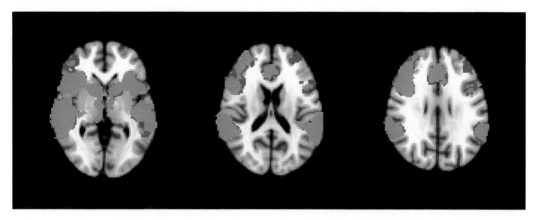

Figure 4.7.   A comparison of activation maps for group analyses using linear registration (FSL FLIRT) versus high-dimensional nonlinear registration (FSL FNIRT), from a group analysis of activation on a stop-signal task. Voxels in red were activated for both analyses, those in green show voxels that were active for linear but not nonlinear registration, and those in blue were active for nonlinear but not for linear registration. There are a number of regions in the lateral prefrontal cortex that were only detected after using nonlinear registration. (Images courtesy of Eliza Congdon, UCLA)

results have not been extensively examined. One study (Ardekani et al., 2004) examined the effects of using registration methods with varying degrees of complexity and found that using high-dimensional nonlinear warping (with the ART package) resulted in greater sensitivity and reproducibility. Figure 4.7 shows the results from a comparison of group analyses performed on data normalized using either affine registration or high-dimensional nonlinear registration. What is evident from this analysis is that there are some regions where smaller clusters of activation are not detected when using affine registration but are detected using high-dimensional registration. At the same time, the significant clusters are smaller in many places for the nonlinear registration, reflecting the fact that better alignment will often result in more precise localization. These results suggest that nonlinear registration is generally preferred over linear registration.

A number of nonlinear registration methods were compared by (Klein et al., 2009), who compared their degree of accuracy by measuring the resulting alignment of anatomical regions using manually labeled brains. They found that the nonlinear algorithms in general outperformed linear registration, but that there was substantial variability between the different packages in their performance, with ART, SYN, IRTK, and DARTEL performing the best across various tests. One notable feature of this study is that the data and code used to run the analyses have been made publicly available at http://www.mindboggle.info/papers/evaluation_NeuroImage2009.php, so that the accuracy of additional methods can be compared to these existing results.

4.10 Quality control for spatial normalization

It is essential to check the quality of any registration operation, including coregistration and spatial normalization.

One useful step is to examine the normalized image with the outline of the template (or reference image, in the case of coregistration) overlaid on the registered image. This is provided in the registration reports from SPM and FSL (see Figure 4.8) and is potentially the most useful tool because it provides the clearest view of the overlap between images.

Another useful quality control step for spatial normalization is to examine the average of the normalized brains. If the normalization operations have been successful, then the averaged brain should look like a blurry version of a real brain, with the blurriness depending upon the dimensionality of the warp. If the outlines of individual brains are evident in the average, then this also suggests that there may be problems with the normalization of some individuals, and that the normalization should be examined in more detail.

Finally, another useful operation is to view the series of normalized images for each individual as a movie (e.g., using the movie function in FSLview). Any images that were not properly normalized should pop out as being particularly "jumpy" in the movie.

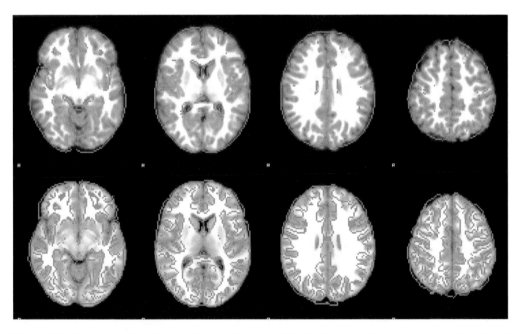

Figure 4.8.   Examples of outline overlays produced by FSL. The top row shows contour outlines from the MNI template overlaid on the subject's anatomical image, whereas the bottom row shows the outlines from the subject's anatomy overlaid on the template. In this case, registration worked relatively well and there is only minor mismatch between the two images.

4.11 Troubleshooting normalization problems

If problems are encountered in the quality control phase, then it is important to debug them. If the problem is a large degree of variation across individuals in the registration, then you should make sure that the template that is being used matches the brain images that are being registered. For example, if the images being registered have been subjected to brain extraction, then the template should also be brain-extracted. Otherwise, the surface of the cortex in the image may be aligned to the surface of the scalp in the template. Another source of systematic problems can come from systematic differences in the orientation of images, which can arise from the conversion of images from scanner formats to standard image formats. Thus, one of the first steps in troubleshooting a systematic misregistration problem should be to make sure that the images being normalized have the same overall orientation as the template. The best way to do this is to view the image in a viewer that shows all three orthogonal directions (saggital, axial, and coronal), and make sure that the planes in both images fall within the same section in the viewer (i.e., that the coronal section appears in the same place in both images). Otherwise, it may be necessary to swap the dimensions of the image to make them match. Switching dimensions should be done with great care, however, to ensure that left/right orientation is not inadvertently changed.

If the problem lies in misregistration of a single individual, then the first step is to make sure that the preprocessing operations (such as brain extraction) were performed successfully. For example, brain extraction methods can sometimes leave large chunks of tissue around the neck, which can result in failed registration. In other cases, misregistration may occur due to errors such as registering an image that has not been brain-extracted to a brain-extracted template (see Figure 4.9). In this case, it may be necessary to rerun the brain extraction using different options or to perform manual editing of the image to remove the offending tissue. If this is not the case, then registration can sometimes be improved by manually reorienting the images so that they are closer to the target image, for example, by manually translating and rotating the image so that it better aligns to the template image prior to registration.

4.12 Normalizing data from special populations

There is increasing interest in using fMRI to understand the changes in brain function that occur with brain development, aging, and brain disorders. However, both aging and development are also associated with changes in brain structure, which can make it difficult to align the brains of individuals at different ages. Figure 4.10 shows examples of brains from individuals across the lifespan, to highlight how different their brain structures can be. These problems are ever greater when examining patients with brain lesions (e.g., due to strokes or tumors). Fortunately, there are methods to address each of these problems.

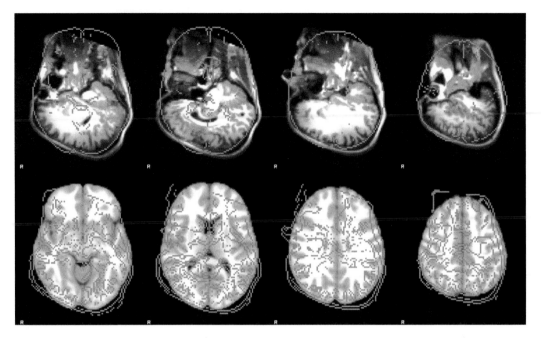

Figure 4.9.   An example of failed registration, in this case due to registering an image that was not brain-extracted to a brain-extracted template.

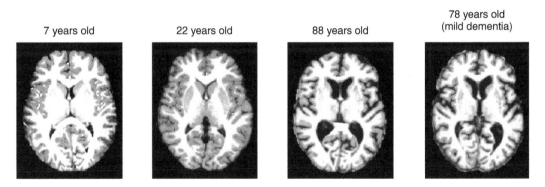

| 7 years old | 22 years old | 88 years old | 78 years old (mild dementia) |

Figure 4.10. Example slices from spatially normalized images obtained from four individuals: a 7-year-old child, a 22-year-old adult, a healthy 88-year-old adult, and a 78-year-old adult with mild dementia. Adult images obtained from OASIS cross-sectional dataset (Marcus et al., 2007).

4.12.1 Normalizing data from children

The child's brain exhibits massive changes over the first decade of life. Not only does the size and shape of the brain change, but in addition there is ongoing myelination of the white matter, which changes the relative MRI contrast of gray and white matter. By about age 7 the human brain reaches 95% of its adult size (Caviness et al.,

1996), but maturational changes in brain structure, such as cortical thickness and myelination, continue well into young adulthood. To compare fMRI data between children and adults, it is necessary to use a spatial normalization method that either explicitly accounts for these changes or is robust to them.

One way to explicitly account for age-related changes is to normalize to a pediatric template (Wilke et al., 2002), or even to an age-specific template. The use of age-specific templates will likely improve registration within the subject group. However, we would caution against using age-specific templates in studies that wish to compare between ages, because the use of different templates for different groups is likely to result in systematic misregistration between groups.

Fortunately, common normalization methods have been shown to be relatively robust to age-related differences in brain structure, at least for children of 7 years and older. Burgund et al. (2002) examined the spatial error that occurred when the brains of children and adults were warped to an adult template using affine registration. They found that there were small but systematic errors of registration between children and adults, on the order of about 5 mm. However, they showed using simulated data that errors of this magnitude did not result in spurious differences in fMRI activation between groups. Thus, for developmental studies that compare activation between individuals of different ages, normalizing to a common template seems to be a reasonable approach.

4.12.2 Normalizing data from the elderly

Normalizing data from elderly individuals poses another set of challenges (Samanez-Larkin & D'Esposito, 2008). Aging is associated with decrease in gray matter volume and increase in the volume of cerebrospinal fluid, as well as an increase in variability across individuals. Further, a nonnegligible proportion of the aged population will suffer from brain degeneration due to diseases such as Alzheimer's disease or cerebrovascular disorders, resulting in marked brain atrophy. The potential problems in normalization arising from these issues suggest that quality control is even more important when working with data from older individuals. One approach that has been suggested is the use of custom templates that are matched to the age of the group being studied (Buckner et al., 2004). The availability of large image databases, such as the OASIS database (Marcus et al., 2007), make this possible, but there are several caveats. First, the custom template should be derived from images that use the same MRI pulse sequence as the data being studied. Second, it is important to keep in mind that although group results may be better when using a custom population-specific template, the resulting coordinates may not match well to the standard space. One potential solution to this problem is to directly compare the custom atlas to an MNI atlas, as demonstrated by Lancaster et al. (2007).

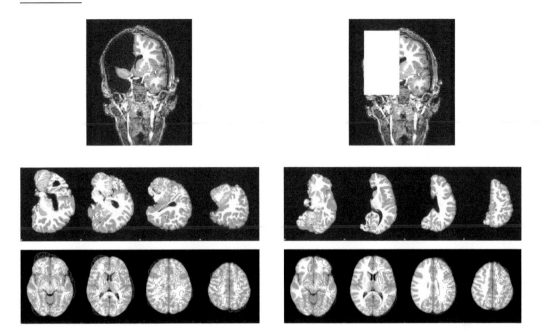

Figure 4.11. An example of the use of cost function masking to improve registration in the presence of lesions. The data used here are from an individual who underwent a right hemispherectomy, and thus is missing most of the tissue in the right hemisphere. The top left panel shows the MRI for this subject, which has a large area of missing signal in the right hemisphere. The lower left panels show the result of spatial normalization using this original image; the registration failed, with serious misalignment between the registered brain (shown in the second row) and the template (shown in the third row with the outline of the registered image). The top right panel shows the cost function mask that was created to mask out the lesioned area (in white). The bottom right panels show the results of successful registration using this cost function mask to exclude this region.

4.12.3 Normalizing data with lesions

Brain lesions can lead to large regions of missing signal in the anatomical image, which can result in substantial errors in spatial normalization (see Figure 4.11). The standard way to deal with this problem is to use *cost function masking*, in which a portion of the image (usually corresponding to the lesion location) is excluded from the cost function computation during registration (Brett et al., 2001). Thus, the normalization solution can be driven only by the good portions of the image. However, it is important to keep in mind that the effects of a lesion often extend beyond the lesion itself, for example, by pushing on nearby regions. If this distortion of other regions is serious enough, then it is likely to be impossible to accurately normalize the image. In this case, an approach using anatomically based regions of interest may be the best way to aggregate across subjects.

## 5

Statistical modeling: Single subject analysis

The goal of an fMRI data analysis is to analyze each voxel's time series to see whether the BOLD signal changes in response to some manipulation. For example, if a stimulus was repeatedly presented to a subject in a blocked fashion, following the trend shown in the red line in the top panel of Figure 5.1, we would search for voxel time series that match this pattern, such as the BOLD signal shown in blue. The tool used to fit and detect this variation is the general linear model (GLM), where the BOLD time series plays the role of dependent variable, and the independent variables in the model reflect the expected BOLD stimulus timecourses. Observe, though, that square wave predictor in red doesn't follow the BOLD data very well, due to sluggish response of the physiology. This leads to one major focus of this chapter: Using our understanding of the BOLD response to create GLM predictors that will model the BOLD signal as accurately as possible. The other focus is modeling and accounting for BOLD noise and other souces of variation in fMRI time series.

Throughout this chapter the models being discussed will refer to modeling the BOLD signal in a single voxel in the brain. Such a voxel-by-voxel approach is known as a mass univariate data analysis, in contrast to a multivariate approach (see Chapters 8 and 9 for uses of multivariate models). We assume that the reader has a basic understanding of the general linear model; for a review see Appendix A. Once the data in all of the voxels are analyzed separately, they are combined across subjects for a group analysis (as described in Chapter 6) and then the statistics are assessed as an image as part of inference (as described in Chapter 7).

5.1 The BOLD signal

As described in Chapter 1, the BOLD signal arises from the interplay of blood flow, blood volume, and blood oxygenation in response to changes in neuronal activity. In short, under an active state, the local concentration of oxygenated hemoglobin increases, which increases homogeneity of magnetic susceptibility, resulting in an

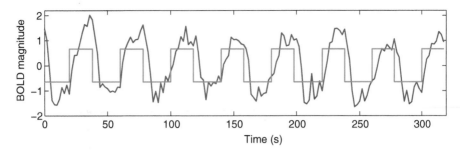

Figure 5.1.   Illustration of BOLD fMRI time series in active voxel and illustration of an unconvolved signal used to model the signal. The BOLD signal for an active voxel (blue) and the stimulus time series (red) is shown.

increase in T2*-weighted MRI signal. As shown in Figure 5.1 the BOLD signal (blue) does not increase instantaneously and does not return to baseline immediately after the stimulus ends (red). Because these changes in blood flow are relatively slow (evolving over several seconds), the BOLD signal is a blurred and delayed representation of the original neural signal.

The hemodynamic response can be described as the ideal, noiseless response to an infinitesimally brief stimulus. It has a number of important characteristics, shown in Figure 5.2:

- **Peak height:** This is the most common feature of interest, since it is most directly related to the amount of neuronal activity in the tissue (Logothetis et al., 2001). For BOLD fMRI, the maximum observed amplitude is about 5% for primary sensory stimulation, whereas signals of interest in cognitive studies are often in the 0.1–0.5% range.
- **Time to peak:** The peak of the HRF generally falls within 4–6 seconds of the stimulus onset.
- **Width:** The HRF rises within 1–2 seconds and returns to baseline by 12–20 seconds after the stimulus onset.
- **Initial dip:** Some studies have identified an initial dip in the BOLD signal that occurs within the first 1–2 seconds and is thought to reflect early oxygen consumption before changes in blood flow and volume occur (Buxton, 2001). Many studies have not found the initial dip, and when it is observed, it is generally a very small signal in comparison to the peak positive BOLD response. It is generally ignored in most models of fMRI data.
- **Poststimulus undershoot:** The HRF generally shows a late undershoot, which is relatively small in amplitude compared to the positive response and persists up to 20 seconds or more after the stimulus.

Importantly, there is substantial variability in each of these features of the HRF across brain areas and across individuals. For example, in the work of Kruggel & von Cramon (1999), the time until peak varied between 6 and 11 seconds across

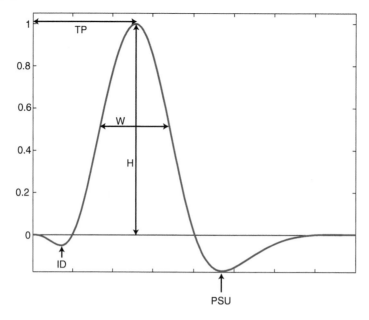

Figure 5.2.   Characteristics of the hemodynamic response. The shape of the HRF function can be described by a variety of characteristics including the time from the stimulus until peak (*TP*), height of response (*H*), the width of the HRF at half the height (*W*), poststimulus undershoot (*PSU*) and in some cases an initial dip (*ID*).

voxels in a single subject. In Handwerker et al. (2004), a study of the HRF shape revealed that both the time until peak and width of the HRF varied within subjects across different regions of the brain and across subjects, with intersubject variability higher than intrasubject variability. And D'Esposito et al. (2003) reviewed a number of studies that compared the BOLD response in healthy young and eldery subjects and found, while the shape of the HRF was simlar between the groups, elderly had reduced signal-to-noise ratios in the response magnitudes.

5.1.1 Convolution

An important characteristic of the BOLD signal is that the relationship between the neural response and the BOLD signal exhibits *linear time invariant* (LTI) properties. The meaning of *linearity* is that if a neural response is scaled by a factor of a, then the BOLD response is also scaled by this same factor of a. As shown in panel A of Figure 5.3, when the neural response (red) is doubled in magnitude, the expected BOLD response (blue) would then be doubled in magnitude. Linearity also implies additivity, in that if you know what the response is for two separate events, if the events were to both occur close together in time, the resulting signal would be the sum of the independent signals. This is illustrated in panel B of Figure 5.3, where neural responses for separate events (green) add linearly to create the expected BOLD response. *Time invariant* means that if a stimulus is shifted by t seconds, the BOLD response will also be shifted by this same amount.

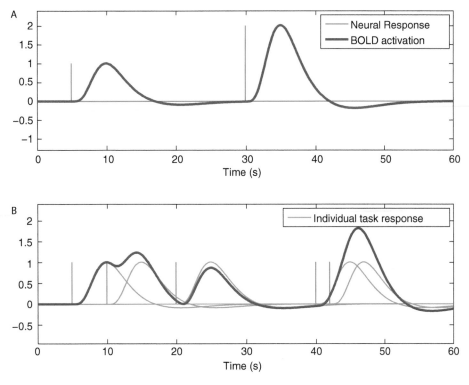

Figure 5.3. Examples of linear time invariance. Panel A illustrates that when a neural signal is twice another, the resulting BOLD activation is also twice as large. Panel B shows how the signals for separate trials, shown in green, add linearly to get the BOLD activation.

Box 5.1.1 What is linear about the hemodynamic response?

The GLM approach to fMRI analysis relies crucially on the assumption that the hemodynamic response is a linear transformation of the underlying neuronal signal, and the question of linearity has been examined in detail in the fMRI literature.

It is first important to point out that there are two possible sources of non-linearity between stimulation and BOLD responses. There could be nonlinearity between the BOLD response and the neuronal signal, which is the main focus of our review here. However, it is well known that there can also be nonlinearities in the relationship between stimuli and neuronal responses. A striking example occurs in the auditory system, where sustained trains of sounds exceeding a particular frequency are associated not with sustained neuronal activity but rather with phasic bursts of activity at the onset and offset of the train (Harms & Melcher, 2002). In other cases, such nonlinearities can occur due to

---

Box 5.1.1 (Continued)

neuronal adaptation, whereby the neuronal response to the same stimulus becomes decreased upon repetition of that stimulus. Thus, it is always important to take into account known neurophysiological data when devising models for fMRI studies.

In early work by Dale & Buckner (1997), stimuli were presented in rapid succession and the assumption of linearity was tested by examining whether the estimated response to multiple stimuli matched the response to a single stimulus. This work showed that the response was indeed largely linear, and that the estimated hemodynamic responses to subsequent trials were very similar to the responses to a single trial. However, this match was not exact; in particular, the estimates on subsequent trials were somewhat compressed relative to the first trial. Further work has confirmed this nonlinearity, particularly for stimuli that occur less than 2 seconds apart (e.g., Wager et al., 2005). Another nonlinearity that has been noted relates to stimulus duration, whereby very brief stimuli exhibit much larger BOLD responses than would be expected based on longer stimuli. For example, Yeşilyurt et al. (2008) found that the BOLD response to a 5-millisecond visual stimulus was only half as large as the response to a 1,000-millisecond stimulus. Fortunately, while these nonlinearities are clearly important, for the range in which most cognitive fMRI studies occur, they will have relatively small impact.

The LTI properties of the BOLD signal have been studied in detail (see Box 5.1.1.), and there is a general consensus that the transform from neuronal activity to BOLD signal is largely LTI. Because of this, a natural approach to creating an expected BOLD signal from a given neural input is to use the convolution operation. Convolution is a way of blending two functions together in an LTI fashion. Specifically, the stimulus onset time series, f (such as the red trend in Figure 5.1) is blended with an HRF, h, creating a shape that more closely represents the shape of the BOLD response. The operation is given by

$$(h * f)(t) = \int h(\tau)f(t - \tau)d\tau \qquad (5.1)$$

Recall that in Section 3.7 convolution was used in a slightly different context when data were *spatially* smoothed by convolving the data with a Gaussian kernel.

Choosing an appropriate HRF function is key in capturing the shape as best as possible and will ensure a good fit of the GLM regressors to the BOLD time series when signal is present.

5.1.1.1 Characterizing the hemodynamic response function

To obtain the predicted BOLD response using convolution, we need an estimate of the HRF. One way to estimate the shape of the response is to present stimuli that are

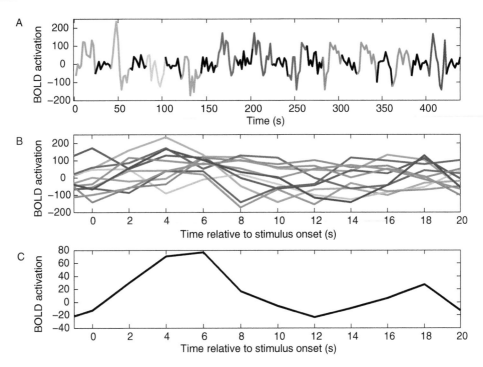

Figure 5.4.   Example of selective averaging. Panel A shows the original time series, highlighting the 22-second window around each stimulus presentation. Panel B overlays the windowed BOLD time series, and panel C shows the average of the windowed time series.

widely spaced in time (e.g., every 30 seconds) and then simply to average the evoked responses at each point in time with respect to the stimulus (referred to variously as *peristimulus time averaging, selective averaging,* or *deconvolution*). Figure 5.4 shows an example of such a process. Panel A shows the original time series, where 22-second windows around each stimulus (starting 2 seconds before the stimulus and lasting for 20 seconds after) are highlighted in different colors. The 11 windowed segments are overlaid in panel B and after averaging the timecourses (panel C) a less noisy image of the response function is obtained.

The work of Friston et al. (1994a) and Lange & Zeger (1997) applied deconvolution models to BOLD data to characterize the HRF and found that, in general, it was approximately described by a gamma function. The choice of the "canonical" HRF using a single gamma function was common until it was realized that the model fit could be further improved by accounting for the poststimulus undershoot, which is not modeled with a single gamma HRF. For this reason, a canonical HRF based on the combination of two gamma functions, known as a *double-gamma HRF*, was adopted (Friston et al., 1998; Glover, 1999). The first gamma function models the shape of the initial stimulus response and the second gamma function models the undershoot. Each analysis software package has default parameter settings that generate a

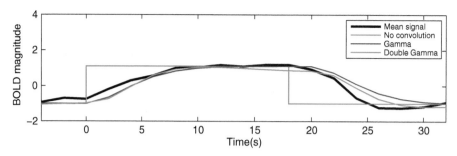

Figure 5.5.   Illustration of different canonical hemodynamic response functions. The black line is the average BOLD response over multiple presentations of a block of stimuli. The red line is the unconvolved time course, blue uses the gamma HRF, whereas the green line is the double gamma, which fits the data best as it accounts for the poststimulus undershoot.

canonical HRF. For example, the default double gamma HRF in SPM has a delay of response set to 6 seconds and a delay of undershoot (relative to onset) of 16 seconds, among five other parameters. These defaults are used in all analyses unless specified otherwise by the user. The only parameter that is free to vary, which is actually estimated in the linear model, is the height of the response. Figure 5.5 illustrates the model fit to data (black) for the boxcar regressor (red), boxcar convolved with a gamma HRF (blue), and boxcar convolved with a double gamma HRF (green). The double gamma has a better fit, since it models the poststimulus undershoot. If a gamma is used instead of a double gamma when there is a strong poststimulus undershoot, the undershoot may pull down the baseline of the model, and as a result the height of the response may be underestimated.

5.1.2 Beyond the canonical HRF

The approach described previously assumed that the HRF could be accurately described using a single canonical response function. However, as was seen in Figure 1.2, hemodynamic responses may differ substantially between individuals in their shape, time to peak, and other aspects. In addition, a number of studies have shown that the shape of the hemodynamic response also differs across different brain regions for the same individual. If we use the canonical HRF, then we are biased to only find responses that are similar to that function. On the other hand, if we use a more complicated model allowing for more flexibility in the shape of the HRF by incorporating more parameters, we will have more variability in the estimates. This is what is often referred to as the *bias-variance tradeoff*. Because of the known variability in the HRF, it is common to use more complicated and flexible models in fMRI analysis.

If we do need a more flexible HRF model, there are a number of approaches that can be used to capture a broader range of response profiles. A popular approach is to use a set of HRF basis functions, functions that when combined linearly give a range of expected shapes for the hemodynamic response. Using just the single canonical response function is the special case of using just one basis function. A two basis function example is the use of a single canonical response function as well as its derivative, allowing for a slight temporal shift. Some early work modeling fMRI data used Fourier sets (or sets of sine and cosine functions) to model the hemodynamic response (Josephs et al., 1997). Other basis sets include the *finite impulse response model* (FIR) set and constrained basis sets. We now review each of these approaches in turn.

5.1.2.1 Modeling the derivative

Probably the most commonly used basis set for fMRI analysis is the "canonical HRF plus derivatives" approach developed by Friston et al. (1998). The rationale for including the temporal derivative is that this basis can capture small offsets in the time to peak of the response. Given the expected signal, $Y(t) = \beta X(t)$, a time-shifted version of the hemodynamic response function can be described as $Y(t) = \beta X(t + \delta)$. However, the shift δ is not linear and hence cannot be estimated with the GLM. However, a Taylor series expansion of $X(t + \delta)$ with respect to δ gives a linear approximation, $Y(t) = \beta(X(t) + \delta X'(t) + \cdots)$, implying a GLM of $Y(t) \approx \beta_1 X(t) + \beta_2 X'(t)$. The β_2 term is not directly interpretable as a delay parameter, but linear combinations of $X(t)$ and $X'(t)$ will model small time shifts of the HRF. Figure 5.6 shows the standard regressor, consisting of the convolution of the stimulus onset and the canonical HRF, its first derivative and the sum of the two, illustrating how adding the two results in a slight shift to the left.

The same Taylor series approach can be taken with respect to other parameters that describe the canonical HRF. For example, the SPM software offers to include "time & dispersion" derivatives. In this case, a third HRF basis is used that is the derivative of $X(t)$ with respect to width of the response (parameter W shown in

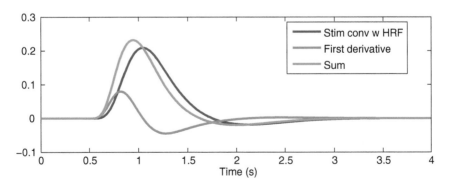

Figure 5.6. The stimulus convolved with the HRF (blue), its derivative (red), and the sum of the two (green), illustrating that including a derivative term in your linear model can adjust for small shifts in the timing of the stimulus.

Figure 5.2). Similar to a temporal derivative that models temporal shifts, this allows the width of the fitted HRF to vary slightly from the canonical HRF.

5.1.2.2 Finite impulse response models

The most flexible model for capturing the HRF shape for a response is the FIR basis set. In this approach, a window around the stimulus is chosen and the GLM is used to model the response at each time point within this window. Figure 5.7 shows an example for a study where one trial type was present, where the left side of the figure illustrates the model and the right panel shows how the parameter estimates from the model reveal the HRF shape. Each regressor models a specific time point in the window surrounding the trial presentation (often called *peristimulus time*). In this case the first regressor corresponds to 2 seconds prior to stimulus presentation, the second is during the stimulus presentation and so on, continuing until 20 seconds after the trial onset. Note that in some cases a single time point (row of the design matrix) may be modeled by two different parameters when trials are sufficiently close in time. For example, in this design the first two time points of a trial window overlap with the last two time points of the previous trial window. The GLM will appropriately account for this overlap by virtue of the additivity of the BOLD response.

The flexibility of the FIR model to capture the shape of the HRF comes at the cost of an increase in the variability of the estimates (i.e., a bias–variance tradeoff). While we are less biased about the shape of the HRF, the variability of our estimates

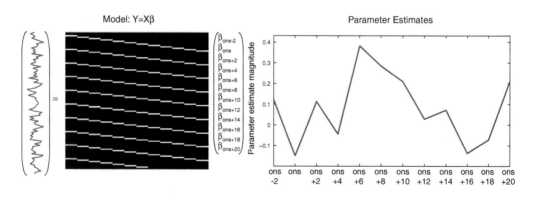

Figure 5.7.   Model and estimates corresponding to an FIR model. On the left is the model used to estimate the FIR parameters, where the BOLD time series is the outcome, the design matrix consists of 0s (black) and 1s (white), and there is a separate parameter estimated for each point in the window around the stimulus. For example, the first regressor and parameter (β_{ons-2}) correspond to the time point 2 seconds prior to onset time, the second regressor is during onset and so on. The *TR* in this case is 2 seconds, so the regressors differ by increments of 2 seconds. The right panel illustrates how the parameter estimates from the FIR model capture the shape of the HRF.

increases since fewer data points are contributing to each parameter's estimate. Additionally, collinearity between the regressors, due to overlapping stimuli, can increase the variability of the estimates further.

One consideration when using the FIR model is how the results of the model fit are used at the next level of analysis. It is common for researchers to fit an FIR model to their data, with reasoning like "I don't want to assume a shape of the hemodynamic response." This is true, but it only holds if one actually uses the entirety of the FIR fit in the higher-level analysis. As discussed in Chapter 6, the standard group modeling approach assumes the data have been distilled down to one BOLD measure per subject (e.g., the parmeter for an event modeled with a canonical HRF). However, a FIR fit consists of many measures (e.g., 12 values in the example in Figure 5.7), and this requires a type of multivariate model to fit all of these responses at the group level. Some authors simply select the parameter from a single FIR bin to take to a group analysis, however this itself implies an assumption that the peak BOLD response falls at that time point. In general, FIR models are most appropriate for studies focused on the characterization of the shape of the hemodynamic response, and not for studies that are primarily focused on detecting activation.

5.1.2.3 Constrained basis sets

At one end of the spectrum there is the lower-bias, higher-variance FIR basis set and at the other end is the higher-bias, lower-variance canonical HRF basis function. An approach that falls somewhere in the middle of the bias–variance spectrum is the use of constrained basis sets, which takes into account known features of the hemodynamic response (such as the fact that it is smooth, starts at zero, ramps slowly, and returns to zero) but still allows flexibility to fit a range of possible responses. Instead of convolving the stimulus onset time series with a single canonical HRF, a set of functions that capture different aspects of the shape of the HRF are used. One approach to constructing a set of basis functions is to first generate a set of HRF shapes that are reasonable, say by varying some of the parameters outlined in Figure 5.2, and then using principal components analysis to extract a set of basis functions that describe this set well. This is the approach taken by Woolrich et al. (2004a) in the FMIRB Linear Optimal Basis Set (FLOBS) algorithm. Figure 5.8 shows an example of four-function basis set developed using this approach (panel A), and some examples of HRF shapes that can be created using linear combinations of these functions (panel B). Although some shape is imposed, different linear combinations of these shapes allow for a larger variety of HRF shapes than using a single canonical basis function.

The benefit of this basis set is that instead of the, say, 12 parameters that must be estimated for the FIR model, only 4 parameters must be estimated for this basis set, which helps reduce the variability of the estimates. Figure 5.9 illustrates the fit of three approaches: double gamma canonical HRF (blue), a basis set with four basis functions (red), and the FIR model (green). The canonical HRF model is fitting a

A   B

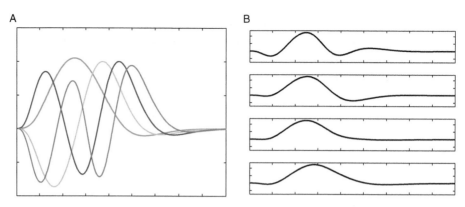

Figure 5.8. Examples of constrained basis sets (panel A) and linear combinations of the basis (panel B). The four basis functions in panel A were produced using the FMRIB linear optimal basis set algorithm. These functions would be convolved with the stimulus onset to create four regressors for modeling the overall HRF shape, compared with the ten regressors shown in the FIR model in Figure 5.7. The right panel illustrates 4 different linear combinations of the basis functions, illustrating the variations in HRF shape that the basis functions are able to model.

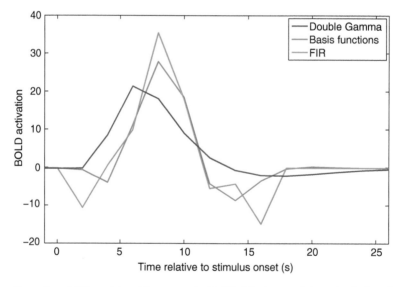

Figure 5.9. Examples of fitting data with a canonical HRF (blue), set of three basis functions (red) and FIR model with ten time points (green). In this case the peak of the double gamma seems to be too early compared to the fits of the more flexible basis function and FIR models. The double gamma fit is smoothest while the FIR model fit is the noisiest.

single parameter and has the smoothest fit, whereas the ten-parameter FIR fit is the noisiest. Both the FIR and four-basis function models illustrate that the imposed time to peak of the double gamma function may be a bit too early and therefore the peak amplitude is underestimated.

In summary, although it would seem that we always want unbiased estimates, often accepting a small amount of bias will result in a greater reduction in variance, especially when that bias fits with our preexisting knowledge about the underlying data. When using models with a large set of basis functions, we must be aware that the flexibility of the model may fit unrealistic HRFs, for example, a shape with two separate positive bumps. In fMRI this means that we usually accept imperfect fit of the canonical HRF in exchange for greater precision and interpretability in our parameter estimates.

5.1.3 Other modeling considerations

Time resolution of the model. The canonical HRF is usually plotted as a smooth curve, as in Figure 5.2, with very fine time resolution. In practice, BOLD time series have time resolution (i.e., repetition time or TR) of 2–3 seconds, yet the events do not usually fall exactly at the begining of an image acquisition nor last the entire *TR*. At coarse time resolution, the stimulus time course for any event or combination of events occurring within the time frame of a single *TR* would look the same at a time resolution of TR seconds, the convolved signal would look the same. For example, if the *TR* = 3 seconds, the following four types of trial presentations would have the same representation at the time resolution of 3 seconds: a stimulus starting at 0 second and lasting 1 second, a stimulus starting at 0 second lasting 2 seconds, a stimulus starting at 0 second and lasting 3 seconds, and a stimulus starting at 2 seconds lasting 1 second. Specifically, the convolved signal for all four of these tasks in a space with a single unit time resolution of 3 seconds would be the dashed black line shown in the right panel of Figure 5.10.

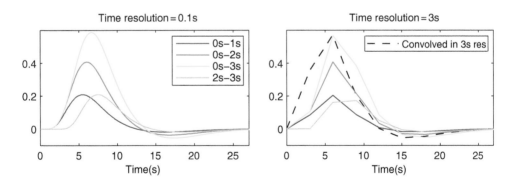

Figure 5.10. Illustrating why convolution is performed in a higher-resolution time domain than the TR. The left panel shows different stimuli, with timings indicated in the legend, convolved with the double gamma HRF in a high-resolution time domain. The right panel illustrates the result that would be acquired for all four stimuli if convolution was done in the lower time resolution of 3 seconds (black dashed line) compared to the signals that are acquired by down-sampling the higher-resolution signals from the left-hand panel (solid colored lines).

To more accurately model the predicted HRF, most software packages first up-sample the stimulus presentation times into a higher time resolution, convolve them with the HRF, and then down-sample the convolved functions to the original time resolution. By doing so, the timing of the stimuli is more accurately represented and since a higher resolution HRF is used, the shape of the response is more accurate. The left-hand side of Figure 5.10 shows the four time courses described previously, convolved in a high time resolution space of 0.1 second. The right panel of the figure shows the down-sampled versions of the time series (solid lines) as well as the signal that would result if the convolution was done in the 3-seconds time resolution space (dotted line). The reason the dotted black line does not match the 3-second event (yellow line) is a result of differences in accuracies of HRF shapes in the two time domains.

Modeling parametric modulation. In many cases, some feature of a stimulus or task can be parametrically varied, with the expectation that this will be reflected in the strength of the neural response. For example, Boynton et al. (1996) parametrically modulated the contrast of a visual stimulus, and showed that neural responses in area V1 responded linearly to this modulation. In designs like this, the parametric modulation can be modeled using an additional regressor in the design matrix, known as a *parametric regressor*. A stimulus onset time series consists of stick functions, usually of equal height. To create a parametric regressor, each onset's stick function has a height reflecting the strength of the stimulus for that trial. Figure 5.11 shows an example of how a parametrically modulated regressor is created. The top panel shows the timing of the stimuli, where the numbers above the stimuli refer to the modulation value. The unmodulated regressor is shown in panel B and panel C shows the modulated version. It is important that the height values are demeaned prior to creating the regressor, in order to ensure that the parametric regressor is not correlated with the unmodulated regressor. It is also important that the GLM always include an unmodulated regressor in addition to the parametrically modulated regressor. This is analogous to the need to include an intercept term in a linear regression model along with the slope term, since without an intercept it is assumed that the fitted line will go through the origin.

Modeling behavioral response times. Historically, most fMRI researchers have not taken response times of the subject's behavioral responses into account in modeling fMRI data; instead, they have used a constant-duration impulse for all trials. However, one of the general maxims of good statistical modeling practice is that if we know of a factor that could affect the data, we should include it in the model. Due to linearity of the BOLD response, we know that twice the neural response results in a BOLD signal that has twice the magnitude. However, as shown in Figure 5.10 a stimulus that is twice as long will also have a BOLD response that is about twice as high (red versus blue line). Thus, trials with longer processing times could have

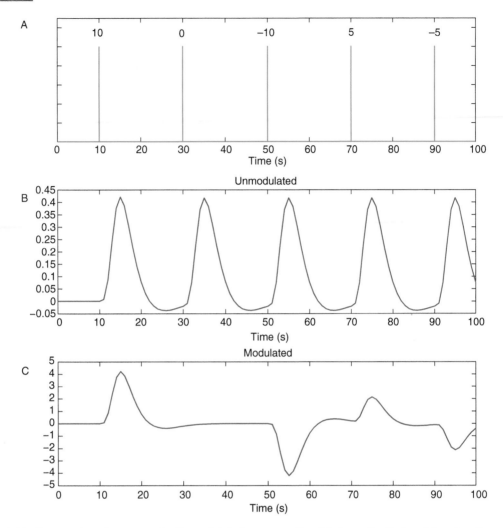

Figure 5.11. Construction of a parametrically modulated regressor. Panel A shows the timing of the stimuli, where the numbers above the stimuli correspond to the modulation value for that stimulus. Panel B shows the unmodulated regressor, and Panel C shows the modulated regressor. Note that both the modulated and unmodulated regressors would be included in the linear regression model.

much greater activation simply due to the amount of time on the task, rather than reflecting any qualitative difference in the nature of neural processing. In fact, it is likely that many differences in activation between conditions observed in functional neuroimaging studies are due simply to the fact that one condition takes longer than the other.

One alternative (recommended by Grinband et al., 2008) is to create the primary regressors in the model using the actual duration of each trial, rather than a fixed duration across trials. This will increase sensitivity for effects that vary with response time but will decrease sensitivity for effects that are constant across trials. A second alternative, which we prefer, is to create the primary regressor using a constant duration, but then include an additional parametric regressor that varies according to response time. This will ensure that the effects of response time are removed from the model and also allows the separate interrogation of constant effects and effects that vary with response time.

Modeling motion parameters.   As described in Section 3.6, head motion during the scan can cause artifacts in the data even after applying image registration methods. As a result, it is a good idea to include motion regressors in the model to account for artifacts and motion-related variance. This is done by including the six time courses of the translation and rotation parameters as *nuisance* regressors in the model. The term nuisance is used to describe regressors that are included in the model to pick up extra variability in the data when there is no interest in carrying out inference on the corresponding parameters. Additionally, it is often beneficial to include the derivatives of the motion parameters, as they can help model motion-related noise and spikes in the data.

Generally we expect that the inclusion of motion regressors will reduce error variance and improve detection power. However, if the motion is correlated with the task, inclusion of the motion regressors may eliminate significant regions seen otherwise. This is because the GLM bases the significance of experimental effects only on the variability uniquely attributable to experimental sources. When such variability is indistinguishable between motion and experimental sources, the significance of the results is reduced, which prevents movement-induced false positives.

Orthogonalization.   A common occurrence in fMRI studies is to have a design that includes regressors that are correlated with each other to some extent. For example, if you were modeling the presentation of a stimulus as well as the subject's response, these two events occur in close proximity, and so the corresponding regressors in the GLM will be highly correlated. The second panel of Figure 5.12 shows an example of correlated regressors ($r = 0.59$), where the green time series represents the stimulus presentation and the red time series models the subject's response 2 seconds later. As just mentioned, the GLM has an essential property in that only the variability unique to a particular regressor drives the parameter estimate for that regressor. The variability described by two regressors X_1 and X_2 can be thought of as having three portions, that unique to X_1, that unique to X_2, and the shared variability. In cases where two regressors are orthogonal (uncorrelated), there is no shared variability component, whereas when they are highly correlated, the unique portion for each regressor is small. This results in unstable and highly variable parameter estimates, which leads to a loss of statistical power.

The data in the top panel of Figure 5.12 contains stimulus- and response-related effects; the second panel of Figure 5.12 shows the model and t-statistics for the

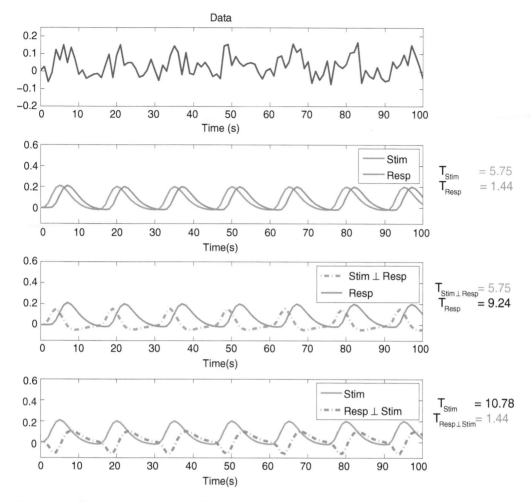

Figure 5.12. Illustration of regressor orthogonalization. The top panel shows simulated data corresponding to a positive response to both the stimulus and response. The second panel shows the highly correlated regressors that would be used to model the stimulus (green) and response (red). The following two panels illustrate what each of the regressors looks like when orthogonalized with respect to the other; the right column shows the t-statistics in each case. Note that the t-statistic for the *non*-orthogonalized regressor is what changes in each case.

model with unaltered simulus and response variables. Even though there is signal, due to correlation between regressors, only one t-statistic is significant. The third panel of Figure 5.12 shows the model after orthogonalizing the stimulus regressor with respect to the response regressor (essentially just the residuals from regressing the red regressor on the green). Now the response t-statistic is very large as we've forced it to take all variation it can; note that the stimulus t-statistic is the same, as its interpretation hasn't changed; it still measures the unique variation attributable to response. The bottom panel of Figure 5.12 shows the reverse situation, after orthogonalizing the response regressor with respect to the stimulus regressor. Now the response t-statistic is very large, and the stimulus regressor's t-statistic matches its original value.

It is because of the arbitrary apportionment of variabilty and signficance just demonstrated that we normally recommend against orthogonalization. Only in cases where variables are clearly serving a supplementary role should orthogonalization be used. For example, when a canonical pluse temporal derivative HRF basis is used, the temporal derivative regressor is orthogonalized with respect to the canonical regressor. This is appropriate because the temporal derivative is only present to reduce error variance, and any shared experimental variance between the two regressors can safely be attributed to the first regressor.

5.2 The BOLD noise

The previous section described how the BOLD signal is modeled, and this section focuses on the other type of variability in the data, the noise. In general the term *noise* is used to describe any variability in the data that is not related to the experimental design. There are two categories of noise. One type is *white noise*, which is broadband and not focused at any particular frequencies. The other, referred to as *structured noise*, reflects coherent sources of variability such as physiological fluctuations that occur at particular frequencies, and thus is *colored* noise. By characterizing the structure of the noise, it can be incorporated into the GLM, improving the fit of the model. Structured noise can result in violations of the assumption of the GLM that observations are not correlated, and false positive rates may increase if it is ignored.

5.2.1 Characterizing the noise

The most obvious characteristic of noise in BOLD fMRI data is the presence of low-frequency drift. Figure 5.13 shows an example of drift in an fMRI time series in both the time domain (left) and the power spectrum in the Fourier domain (right). The power spectrum is acquired by taking the Fourier transform of the time series; the X axis of the plot refers to different frequencies, whereas the Y axis refers to the power, or strength, of this frequency in the data. For example, this voxel is active, and since the frequency of the stimulus is one cycle every 40 seconds, there is a spike in the power spectrum at $1/40$ seconds $= 0.025$ Hz. This time series also exhibits a slowly increasing trend in the time domain, which, since it is low frequency, contributes to the power at lower frequencies of the power spectrum. The shape of the power spectrum is often referred to as the 1/f, or inverse frequency, function (Zarahn et al., 1997).

Initially the source of the 1/f noise structure in fMRI data was not clear. The noise structure was studied in great detail by Aguirre et al. (1997) and Zarahn et al. (1997) in both humans and water phantoms to determine whether the $1/f$ noise was physiologic or due to the scanner. Additionally, they examined a variety of computers and

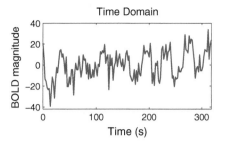 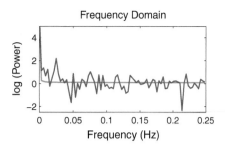

Figure 5.13. Noise structure of fMRI data. The left panel shows the BOLD time series for a voxel that exhibits both signal (blocked pattern is visible) as well as low-frequency drift in the form of a slow uphill trend. The right panel shows the same data in the frequency domain. The red line corresponds to the shape of a fitted $1/f$ function, which matches the shape of the power spectrum well, and the spike in the power spectrum at 0.025 Hz corresponds to the frequency of the task (once every 40 seconds) in this experiment.

equipment to determine whether the $1/f$ noise was due to radiofrequency contamination, but in all cases the $1/f$ structure prevailed. Some of the noise appears to be due to effects of subject movement that remain after motion correction, or cardiac and respiratory effects. However, even when phantoms and cadavers (Smith et al., 1999) are scanned, low-frequency noise persists, indicating that the scanner itself is an additional source of structured noise.

Since low-frequency noise is always present in fMRI data, it is important that when planning a study the frequency of the task does not fall into the range between 0 and 0.015 Hz where the low-frequency noise has typically been found, meaning that the frequency of trial presentation should be faster than one cycle every 65–70 seconds (i.e., a block length of no more than about 35 seconds for an on–off blocked design). If stimuli are grouped together in long blocks, the signal will be lost in the lower frequencies, where the task signal cannot be separated from the noise. If it is necessary to examine effects that change more slowly, one alternative is to use fMRI techniques such as arterial spin labeling (ASL), which do not exhibit such low-frequency fluctuations (e.g., Detre & Wang, 2002).

Removing the low-frequency trends is handled using a combination of two approaches. First, a *high-pass* filter is used to remove low-frequency trends from the data. However, after high-pass filtering, fMRI time series are still correlated over time. As discussed in Appendix A, one assumption of the GLM is that the data are not temporally autocorrelated and that the variance of the data is constant over observations. When these assumptions are violated, the inferences based on the GLM are biased and can result in an elevated false positive rate. Thus, a second step attempts to estimate and undo the correlation structure of the data. The current standard approach is to *prewhiten* the data to remove the temporal autocorrelation, but another approach that was initially considered, *precoloring*, will also be discussed.

5.2.2 High-pass filtering

The most common approach for removing low-frequency trends is to apply what is known as a high-pass filter. One approach of high-pass filtering is to add a discrete cosine transform (DCT) basis set to the design matrix, such as the example shown in Figure 5.14. Figure 5.15 shows the original time series (top) and fit of the DCT basis functions to the data (green). The middle panel shows the original time series (blue) and the high-pass filtered time series using the DCT basis set (green), and the bottom panel shows the same, but in the Fourier domain. After high-pass filtering, the drifting at the beginning and end of the time series is removed. When using a DCT basis set, the highest frequency cosine function that should be included would correspond to the highest frequency that is desired to be removed from the data, which is chosen to avoid the frequency of the experimental task that is also being modeled. As a rough rule of thumb, the longest period of the drift DCT basis should be at least twice the period of an on–off block design.

Another approach to removing the low-frequency drift, which is used by the FSL software package, is to fit a locally weighted scatterplot smoothing, or LOWESS, model to the time series and remove the estimated trend from the data. A LOWESS model fits a local linear regression over a window of the data weighting points in the middle of the window rather than around the edges, for example using a gaussian function as a weight. For details on the LOWESS model, see Cleveland (1979). The result is that the low-frequency trends in the data are picked up by the LOWESS fit, as shown in the top panel of Figure 5.15 (red). After this trend is fit to the data, it is subtracted, resulting in a high-pass filtered data set shown in the middle panel of Figure 5.15. The larger the window, the higher the frequencies that are filtered out of the data, so the window should be chosen to only remove frequencies in the low end of the spectrum far from the frequency of the task. Figure 5.15 shows that in the time domain, the DCT basis function and LOWESS approaches yield very similar results. In the spectral domain, however, the power of the data filtered using the DCT basis set drops to 0 as the frequency decreases, whereas the LOWESS fit has a more gentle roll off as frequency decreases.

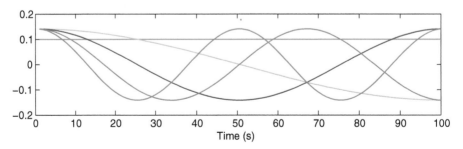

Figure 5.14. Discrete cosine transform basis set. The five lines correspond to the first five discrete cosine transform basis functions, starting with a constant term and then increasing the frequency of the cosine by a half period with each additional curve.

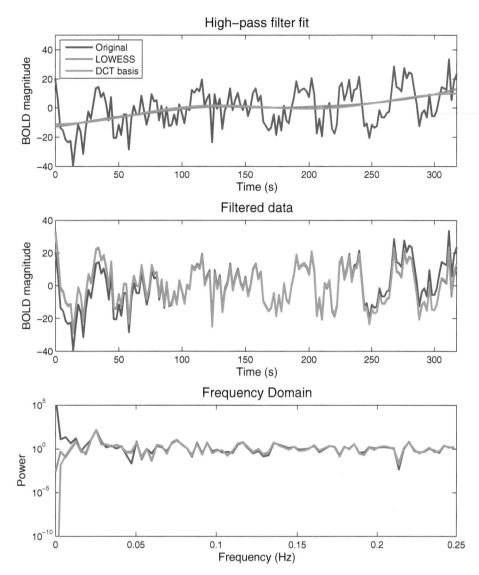

Figure 5.15. Illustration of high-pass filtering. The top panel shows the original time series (blue) as well as the HP filter fit using a LOWESS curve (red) and a DCT basis set (green). In both cases the fit is very similar. The middle panel shows the original data (blue) as well as the filtered data using the two methods. The bottom panel shows the power spectrum of the original data (blue) as well as the filtered data, illustrating that the original time series exhibited low-frequency noise, which is removed by the high-pass filters. Note that the DCT basis set tends to have a sharper decrease at the lowest frequencies, whereas the LOWESS filter has a more gentle roll-off at the edges.

5.2.3 Prewhitening

After high-pass filtering, the fMRI time series are still temporally autocorrelated, where the correlation increases as the temporal proximity of two data points increases. As discussed in Appendix A, in order for the general linear model estimates to be unbiased and have minimum variance among all unbiased estimators, a very appealing quality in an estimate, the data going into the model cannot be correlated, and the variance at each time point must be identical. When data are temporally autocorrelated, prewhitening removes this correlation from the GLM prior to estimation. The prewhitening process is generally carried out in two steps. In the first step, the GLM is fit ignoring temporal autocorrelation to obtain the model residuals, which is the original data with all modeled variability removed. The residuals are then used to estimate the autocorrelation structure, and then model estimation is carried out after prewhitening both the data and the design matrix. In general, the GLM with the original data has the following form:

$$Y = X\boldsymbol{\beta} + \boldsymbol{\epsilon}, \tag{5.2}$$

where Y is the BOLD time series, X is the design matrix, $\boldsymbol{\beta}$ is the vector of parameter estimates, and $\boldsymbol{\epsilon}$ is the error variance, which is assumed to be normally distributed with a mean of 0 and a covariance of $\sigma^2 V$. The GLM estimates for $\boldsymbol{\beta}$ are only optimal when V is the identity matrix, but since the BOLD data are autocorrelated, V is not the identity; it may have nonzero off-diagonal elements representing cross-correlation and may have varying values along the diagonal, representing differences in variance across time. Prewhitening involves finding a matrix, W, such that $WVW' = I_T$, where I_T is an identity matrix with the same number of rows and columns as the time series. Prewhitening involves premultiplying both sides of the GLM by W to give

$$WY = WX\boldsymbol{\beta} + W\epsilon, \tag{5.3}$$

where now the covariance of $W\epsilon$ is $\text{Cov}(W\epsilon) = \sigma^2 WVW' = \sigma^2 I_T$. Therefore, the *whitened* model has independent error terms, and the GLM estimates from this model are optimal. More details can be found in Appendix A.

The reason for using the residuals is so that the prewhitening process only removes temporal autocorrelation present in the data that is *not* related to the task of interest; that is, it removes autocorrelation that is part of the noise rather than part of the signal. Although this process is straightforward, it depends on the model of the temporal autocorrelation being exactly correct. If the correlation is not removed perfectly, the assumptions of the GLM that the data are uncorrelated with equal variance for each time point will be violated, and hence inferences may be biased.

There are different models for BOLD noise that have been found to describe the correlation well. The simplest is known as the $AR(1)$ model and simply assumes the variance of each time point is 1, and the correlation between pairs of data points decreases geometrically as the data are further apart $(\text{cor}(y_i, y_{i+a}) = \rho^a)$. A slightly more complicated correlation model adds an additional variance parameter and is known as the $AR(1)+$ white noise $(AR(1) + WN)$. The added variance is the white noise. This is a special case of a more general correlation model known as the autoregressive, moving average or $ARMA$ model (Box et al., 2008). Specifically the ARMA(1,1), which has one autoregressive parameter like the $AR(1)$ with an additional moving average parameter. All three of these correlation models fit well to the $1/f$ trend found in the power spectra of fMRI time series. Another option is to use an unstructured covariance estimate, where the correlation for each lag in the time series is estimated separately. This tends to have more parameters than the three parameter $AR(1) + WN$, making it less biased, but the correlation estimates are less stable (more variable).

It is important that the correlation model used in fMRI strikes a balance between having enough parameters to describe the correlation structure accurately, but not having too many parameters, since this will cause the estimates to be more variable due to a lack of degrees of freedom. If a modeling approach produces estimates that are too variable, the typical solution to increase the degrees of freedom. Since the degrees of freedom are roughly equal to the number of data points minus the number of parameters being estimated, they can be increased by either increasing the amount of data (e.g., pooling data across multiple voxels) or decreasing the number of parameters being estimated by using a simpler correlation model. One drawback of estimating the temporal autocorrelation model by pooling across multiple voxels is that the temporal autocorrelation structure is not exactly the same for all regions of the brain (Worsley et al., 2002; Zarahn et al., 1997). Likewise, using only a few parameters in the autocorrelation model may not capture the trend thoroughly. All software packages use a combination of both of these tactics. In SPM , for example, a simple $AR(1) + WN$ model is fit globally, pooling information from all voxels found to be significant in a preliminary fit. The model captures the correlation structure well, and by using a global approach, the estimate is not highly variable. FSL, on the other hand, uses a slightly different approach with an unstructured autocorrelation estimate, meaning a nonparametric approach is used to estimate the correlation for each lag of the time series. Instead of having a global estimate of the correlation, FSL instead smoothes the correlation estimate spatially. Additionally, since the correlations for high lags have very few time points, these estimates are highly variable. To solve this issue, FSL uses a Tukey Taper, which smoothes the correlation estimate in the spectral domain to the point where correlations at high lags are set to 0. Typically around 6–12 parameters are used for this voxelwise correlation estimation.

5.2.4 Precoloring

Whether fMRI time series should be whitened or, the opposite, temporally smoothed, was at one point a contentious topic in the fMRI analysis literature. Even though it is theoretically optimal, prewhitening was not commonly used intially. This was in part due to inaccurate correlation models that gave biased variance estimates and could inflate false positive risk (Friston et al., 2000). Temporal smoothing or low-pass filtering, dubbed *precoloring* was initially considered as a better approach to modeling temporal autocorrelation as it did not have the same problems with bias that prewhitening had (prior to the employment of the regularization strategies discussed above).

The general idea behind precoloring is that since we do not know the true structure of the temporal autocorrelation, we impose more autocorrelation with a low-pass filter. While strictly the autocorrelation in the data is now a combination of an unknown intrinsic autocorrelation and the smoothing-induced autocorrelation, the latter swamps the former, and we assume the autocorrelation is known and equal to that from the low-pass filtering. With a known autocorrelation, the standard errors and the degrees of freedom can then be adjusted to eliminate bias and produce valid inferences. Figures 5.16 and 5.17 illustrate all types of filtering for blocked stimuli and random stimuli, respectively. The top panels show the original data in the time (left) and spectral (right) domains, the second and third panels show high-pass and low-pass filtering, and the bottom panel show bandpass filtering, which is both high and low-pass filtering. Bandpass filtering was introduced earlier (Section 2.4.2) in terms of spatial filtering of fMRI data. Just as high-pass filtering the data removes low-frequency trends in the data, low-pass filtering removes high-frequency trends in the data.

The major problem with low-pass filtering the data is that in many fMRI experiments the stimuli are presented in a random fashion, meaning that the signal covers a wide range of frequencies, including some high-frequencies. When data are low-pass filtered, the high-frequency components are removed from the data, which means signal is being removed from the data. As Figure 5.16 shows with a block design, since most of the power for the task is focused at lower frequencies, the high-pass filter does not remove the task-based trends from the data. On the other hand, Figure 5.17 shows that in an event-related study, the power for the task is spread across a wide range of frequencies and so the low-pass filter ends up removing some of the task signal. Because of this and also due to the development of better regularization approaches for prewhitening, precoloring is not a recommended solution for dealing with temporal autocorrelation.

5.3 Study design and modeling strategies

Depending on what the investigator is interested in measuring, different study designs and modeling strategies are required. On one end of the spectrum, the

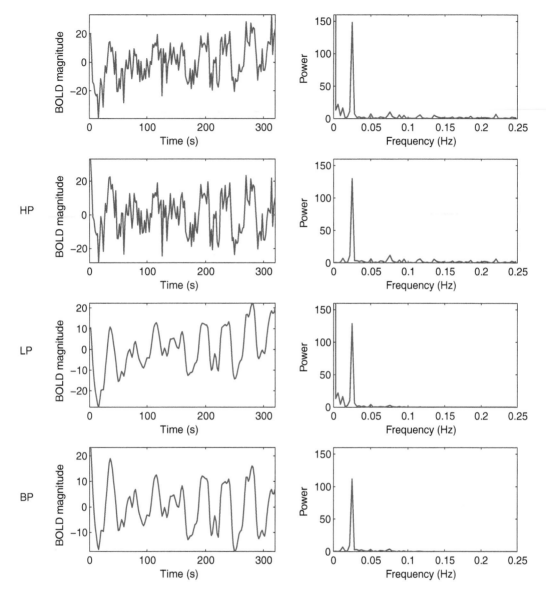

Figure 5.16. Illustration of different filtering approaches on data with blocked trials. The left column shows the result in the time domain, and the right column, in the Fourier domain. The first row is the original data followed by high-pass (HP), low-pass (LP), and bandpass (BP) filtered data, respectively. When trials are blocked, most of the task-based frequency is focused at one point (0.25 Hz in this case), while the rest is aliased to other frequencies. The HP filter removes low-frequency drift, as shown before, whereas the LP filter removes high-frequency trends. Applying both in the BP filtered case removes variability at both low and high frequencies but preserves the bulk of the signal at 0.25 Hz.

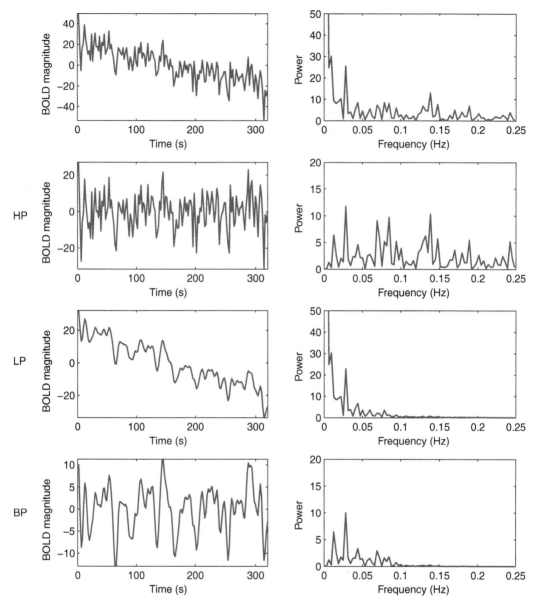

Figure 5.17. Illustration of different filtering approaches on data with randomly spaced trials. The left column shows the result in the time domain, and the right column, in the Fourier domain. The first row is the original data followed by high-pass (HP), low-pass (LP), and bandpass (BP) filtered data, respectively. Since the trials are spaced randomly in time, the task energy is spread over a wide range of higher frequencies. In the LP-filtered case, only low-frequency noise is removed, but in the LP and BP filtered cases, much of the higher frequency signal is removed by the filter, which will have a negative impact on our GLM inferences since there is little signal left to detect.

investigator may only be interested in detecting and estimating the magnitude of activation (referred to as *detection*). On the other hand, the investigator may be interested in estimating the precise shape of the hemodynamic response associated with the task (referred to as *estimation*). Not only are different models required to test each of these hypothesis, but different study designs are more appropriate for testing each; in fact, as we will see later, designs that are optimized to test for one of them will in general be relatively poor at testing the other. Additionally, when multiple task types are present in a study, some study designs are more optimal than others. These issues will be discussed in the following sections.

5.3.1 Study design: Estimation and detection

Imagine you have a small pile of sand on your kitchen floor (the size of a handful). From a distance it is easy to deduce that there is indeed a pile of sand on your floor. If you kneel down and look very closely at the sand without touching it you would be able to see the shapes of some of the granules that were on the outside of the pile, but you cannot study the shape of the granules in the middle. In this case we would say our ability to *detect* the presence of sand was quite high, but our ability to *estimate* the shape of the granules of the sand was not as good. Now imagine that you spread the sand around on the floor with your hand. Once it is spread out, you can look closely and see almost every side of each granule of sand and you can gather more information on the shape of the individual granule. On the other hand, if you stood up and backed away, it would not be as easy to detect that there was sand on the floor and where, specifically, the sand was. So, in this case our ability to estimate the shape is good, but our detection ability is poor.

This analogy can also be applied to trials in an fMRI experiment. If the investigator is mostly concerned with detecting the presence of a response, the best way to ensure this is to block the trials together. Note, when this is done, we only get a little bit of information about the shape of the HRF from the few trials at the beginning and the end of the block, whereas the ones in the middle do not tell us anything about the shape but do contribute to the ability to detect the response. On the other hand, if we separate the trials with a little bit of time, it is much easier to capture the specific shape of the HRF from our data. Note that if the trials have too much time between them and occur at regular intervals, there won't be enough trials to estimate the HRF shape very well, and the study will be very boring for the test subject, which will decrease the quality of the data. The solution is to use randomly spaced trials. The GLM model is able to pick out the shape of the HRF through the FIR model, or other models described in Section 5.1.2, and since more trials are included the estimates will be less variable.

To strike a balance between estimation and detection, one suggestion is to use a semi-random design, which can be constructed by starting with the trials blocked and then randomly moving trials to break up the blocked shape (Liu et al., 2001). It should be noted that if a design has trials that are blocked as well as randomly spaced, the blocked trials should be modeled separate from the spaced trials. This is because the mental processes for separated stimuli may be different than when the stimuli are rapidly presented and so the interpretation of the two types of stimulus presentation differ.

5.3.2 Study design: Multiple stimulus types

The previous section primarily concerns a study where there is only a single type of stimulus presented, but in most cases two or more stimulus or trial types are involved, and then it must be determined what order these stimuli will be presented and how much time will be between each stimulus. In some cases, the order of the stimuli is fixed, for example when a cue is given followed by a stimulus that the subject then responds to, the events always occur in the order of cue, stimulus, response. When regressors in a GLM are highly correlated, the estimates of the parameters are quite unstable and hence highly variable. Another way of stating that an estimate has high variability is to say it has low efficiency. Efficiency is calculated as the inverse of the parameter estimate's variance. In general, if the design matrix is given by $\mathbf{X}$ and if $\boldsymbol{\beta}$ is the vector of parameters to be estimated in the GLM, the covariance of the parameter estimates is given by

$$\text{Cov}\left(\widehat{\boldsymbol{\beta}}\right) = (\mathbf{X}'\mathbf{X})^{-1}\sigma^2 \tag{5.4}$$

where σ^2 is the error variance. (Here we neglect the whitening, but the equation still works if we replace $\mathbf{X}$ with $\mathbf{WX}$.) Design efficiency typically only refers to the variance due to the design, or $(\mathbf{X}'\mathbf{X})^{-1}$, so for a given contrast of parameters, $\mathbf{c}$, the efficiency for that contrast is defined as

$$\text{eff}\left(\mathbf{c}\widehat{\boldsymbol{\beta}}\right) = \frac{1}{\mathbf{c}(\mathbf{X}'\mathbf{X})^{-1}\mathbf{c}'} \tag{5.5}$$

In the simplest case, if there were two parameters in the model and the interest was in the efficiency of the first parameter, β_1 (corresponding to $H_0 : \beta_1 = 0$) and so the contrast would be $\mathbf{c} = [1\ 0]$. There is not a meaningful cutoff for an acceptable level of efficiency, but instead the efficiencies for a variety of models can be estimated and then the most efficient model would be chosen. A measure related to efficiency with a more meaningful cutoff is the *power* of a statistical test. Since this calculation requires knowledge of σ^2, it is more complicated to estimate and isn't necessary if one simply wants to rank designs to choose the most efficient one, since the most efficient design will by default also have the highest power. A more detailed description of statistical power for fMRI studies is given in Chapter 6.

The top panel of Figure 5.18 shows an example of two correlated regressors, where the timing for one stimulus (blue) always occurs 6 seconds prior to the presentation of a second stimulus (green). In this case, the correlation between the two regressors is very high (corr $= -0.61$), meaning the estimates of the parameters corresponding

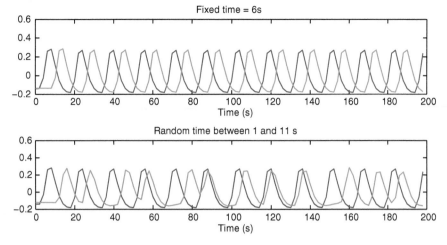

Figure 5.18. How jittering can improve model fit. In the top panel, the time between the first stimulus (blue) and the second (green) is always fixed at 6 seconds, whereas in the bottom panel the time between stimuli is randomly chosen between 1 and 10 seconds (so on average it is 6-seconds). The regressors in the top panel are more highly correlated (corr = −0.61); the correlation between regressors in the bottom panel is much smaller in magnitude (corr = −0.15). As a result, the design in the bottom panel is more efficient at estimating the magnitudes of each stimulus.

to each trial type are highly variable. The value of $(\mathbf{X}'\mathbf{X})^{-1}$ for this fixed ISI design $(\mathbf{X}_F)$ is given by

$$\left(\mathbf{X}_F'\mathbf{X}_F\right)^{-1} = \begin{pmatrix} 0.5632 & 0.3465 \\ 0.3465 & 0.5703 \end{pmatrix} \qquad (5.6)$$

so the efficiency for estimating β_1 (corresponding to the blue stimulus) would be $\frac{1}{0.5632} = 1.76$ and the efficiency for estimating β_2 (corresponding to the green stimulus) is $\frac{1}{0.5703} = 1.75$. In the bottom panel of Figure 5.18, the time between the the first stimulus, and the second stimulus is jittered randomly, where the timing is sampled from a uniform distribution ranging between 1 and 11 seconds. Note, on average, the timing between the first and second trial types is equivalent to what is shown in the top panel (6 seconds). In this case, the correlation between regressors has a smaller magnitude of −0.15, and therefore the estimates for the parameters for each trial type are much less variable. In this case the model variance corresponding to the jittered design, $\mathbf{X}_J$, is given by

$$\left(\mathbf{X}_J'\mathbf{X}_J\right)^{-1} = \begin{pmatrix} 0.3606 & 0.0602 \\ 0.0602 & 0.4640 \end{pmatrix} \qquad (5.7)$$

Note the off-diagonal entries, corresponding to the covariance, are much smaller in this case, and the diagonal elements, corresponding to the variances, are much smaller since there is less collinearity between the regressors. The efficiency for estimating β_1 would be $\frac{1}{0.3606} = 2.77$ and the efficiency for estimating β_2 is $\frac{1}{0.4640} = 2.16$. Compared to the efficiencies of the fixed ISI designs, this random ISI design is 57% more efficient in estimating β_1 and 23% more efficient in estimating β_2. This relates back to the earlier discussion about orthogonality, since in the fixed ISI design regressors are correlated, there is little unique variance for each regressor to be used to estimate the corresponding parameter and hence the efficiency is lower.

5.3.3 Optimizing fMRI designs

When developing a new study design, one must consider a variety of designs and look at both the estimation and detection abilities of those designs and choose the design that is most suitable for the purposes of the study. Additionally, it is important to consider the psychological factors of the experiment. If the ordering of the stimuli is easy to predict there will be problems with habituation of the subject to the task. As more trial types are added to the study the number of possible designs, including different orderings of stimuli and timings between stimuli, is quite large and searching over all designs and checking the estimation and detection abilities of each is not a feasible task. Instead, it is helpful to develop a *search* algorithm that methodically chooses designs. The simplest example of a search algortithm is that of the permuted block design (Liu, 2004). As described earlier, when trials are blocked, the ability to detect the activation corresponding to the blocked stimuli is quite great, but the ability to estimate the shape of the HRF is not great. Additionally, blocked stimuli may not be psychologically interesting for the investigator to study. The permuted block design starts with the stimuli blocked by task type and then TRs are randomly chosen and the stimuli in the TRs are swapped, hence breaking up the blockiness of the design. This is then repeated, and after many iterations the stimuli will be randomly ordered, corresponding to a design where detection has decreased (from the original block design) and estimation of the HRF has increased. Designs along the continuum can be selected for the study, depending on the desired amount of detection and estimation, while keeping the study interesting for the subject.

Another approach to selecting the ordering of stimuli in an experiment is to use what are called maximal length sequences, or M-sequences (Liu & Frank, 2004; Liu, 2004). M-sequences are series of 0s and 1s that are maximally uncorrelated with shifted versions of themselves. Since an FIR model is nothing more than multiple copies of the stimulus stick functions shifted in time, this means that M-sequences will produces FIR models with covariates that have the least amount of correlation between them as possible, which will lead to highly efficient estimates of each lag of the FIR model. This also means that M-sequences are ideal for estimating the shape of the HRF, but not necessarily very good at building designs with high detection power for an assumed canonical HRF.

So far the discussion of optimal designs has not mentioned psychological factors of the design, like predictability and counterbalancing, and other arbitrary constraints on the design, like ensuring that equal number of trials are presented for different trial types. Instead of just optimizing statistical properties, by maximizing a cost function that is a combination of different design "fitness" properties, designs that have good efficiency and psychological properties can be found. The cost function will be quite complicated, however, making traditional optimization methods challenging. This has motivated the use of evolutionary or "genetic algorithms" for finding event-related fMRI designs that maximize arbitrary fitness criterion (Wager & Nichols, 2003). Recent work has improved upon this approach by using M-sequences to find good initial guesses of designs (Kao et al., 2009).

## 6

Statistical modeling: Group analysis

Whereas the previous chapter focused on analyzing the data from a single run for a single subject, this chapter focuses on how we combine the single subject results to obtain group results and test group hypotheses. The most important consideration of the group fMRI model is that it accounts for the so-called repeated measures aspect of the data, which means that subjects are randomly sampled from a larger population, and multiple fMRI measurements are obtained for each subject. If the proper model is not used, inferences will only apply to the particular subjects in the study, as opposed to the population from which they were sampled. In general, it is important that subjects are treated as random effects in the model, which is known as a mixed effects model. The difference between treating subjects as random versus fixed quantities is discussed in the following section.

6.1 The mixed effects model

6.1.1 Motivation

To motivate the need for a mixed effects analysis, we use a simple example from outside of the imaging domain. Instead of measuring brain activity for a subject, imagine that we measure hair length. The goal is to see if there is a difference in the length of hair between men and women and since we clearly cannot measure hair length on all people we randomly sample from the population. Once we know the distributions of hair length for men and women, they can be compared statistically to see if there is a difference.

The experiment begins by randomly selecting four men and four women. Note within each group hair length has two sources of variability: variability of hair length across different hairs from a single person and variability in the length of hair across people due to their different hair cuts. Let σ_W^2 be the within-subject variance and σ_B^2 is between subject variance.

The top eight distributions in Figure 6.1 show the hair length distributions for the four men and four women. Precisely, these distributions describe the relative frequency of hair length of a randomly selected hair from a single individual. Here we have assumed that the variation of a given individual's hair length is 1 inch ($\sigma_W^2 = 1$).

If our population of interest is precisely these eight men and women, then between-subject variation can be neglected, and a fixed effects analysis can be used. Precisely, the question to be answered is: How does the hair length of these *particular* four men compare to that of these *particular* four women? For the sake of illustration, let's assume we sample only a single hair from each subject, for a total of four hairs within each gender group. Then the fixed effects variance of the average hair length in each gender is $\sigma_{FFX}^2 = \frac{1}{4}\sigma_W^2 = 0.25$ inches squared. The resulting fixed effects distributions with variance σ_{FFX}^2, are shown in Figure 6.1, below the individuals' distributions.

Recall that our initial goal was to study the hair length differences between *all* men and *all* women, not just those in our sample as described in the previous paragraph. To extrapolate to the population of all people, we need something that describes the distrubution of hair length across all people. This is accomplished by additionally including the between-subject variance, σ_B^2, which describes the variability of hair length across people. When the between-subject variance is modeled separately from the within-subject variance, it is typically described as treating the subjects as being randomly sampled from the population, or treating the subject as a *random effect*. This type of modeling strategy is more generally referred to as a *mixed model*.

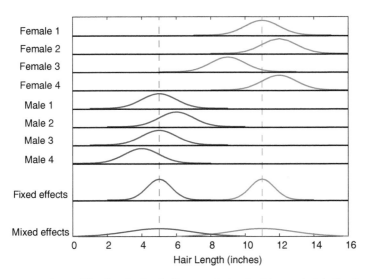

Figure 6.1.   Comparison of fixed and mixed effects analysis. The blue and pink distributions correspond to males and females, respectively. The top eight distributions are subject-specific distributions, followed by the group distributions stemming from fixed effects and mixed effects analysis. The vertical lines indicate the sample means for the two groups.

Assuming $\sigma_B^2 = 49$ inches squared is the between-subject variability in hair length, the total mixed effects variance for each subject is the sum of the two variabilities, $\sigma_W^2 + \sigma_B^2$. Then the total mixed effects variance for the average hair length within each group (again assuming only a single hair has been sample from each subject) is $\sigma_{MFX}^2 = \sigma_W^2/4 + \sigma_B^2/4 = 1/4 + 49/4 = 12.5$. The corresponding mixed effects distribution is shown in the bottom panel of 6.1. Note that if the fixed effects distributions were wrongly used to make a conclusion about all men and women, they would show that males have shorter hair than females, since the distributions have very little overlap. In fact, the mixed effects distributions show considerable overlap, and we would not, based on this small sample, be able to conclude that men and women have different hair length.

One simplification here is that we only measured one hair per person. It would be better to randomly select multiple hairs, measure each, and average. If we instead had measured 25 hairs per person, then the distribution of each subject's average would have variance $\sigma_W^2/25$; for the fixed effect distribution $\sigma_{FFX}^2 = \frac{1}{4}\sigma_W^2/25 = 0.01$ and for the mixed effects distribution $\sigma_{MFX}^2 = \frac{1}{4}\sigma_W^2/25 + \frac{1}{4}\sigma_B^2 = 12.26$. Observe that, since σ_B^2 is so much larger than σ_W^2, increasing intrasubject precision (by sampling more hairs from each individual) has little impact on the mixed effects variance.

Returning to fMRI, the basic issues are essentially the same. Instead of measuring multiple hairs, we are measuring the brain activation at a particular brain location multiple times. In group fMRI studies, most often the interest is in making conclusions about populations and not specific subjects and hence a mixed effects method is necessary to obtain valid inferences from group fMRI data.

6.1.2 Mixed effects modeling approach used in fMRI

The mixed effects model for fMRI is carried out in multiple stages. We will start by assuming that each subject has a single run of fMRI data and that there are multiple subjects. The subjects belong to one of two groups, and the goal of the study is to see whether the activation difference when viewing faces versus houses is different between the two groups (patients and controls). In this case, there are two levels in the model. The first level involves modeling the data for each subject separately; the output of this model is subject-specific estimates of the faces–houses contrast and within-subject variance estimates for this contrast. The left side of Figure 6.2 shows an example of what the first-level model and the corresponding contrasts would look like for testing faces–houses. In these illustrations, it is assumed that the mean of the data and the regressors in the first-level design are 0 and hence an intercept term (column of 1s) is not needed. The second-level model then takes as input the subject-specific parameter estimates and variance estimates from the first-level model. In the example in the right panel Figure 6.2 the group model includes 12 subjects, with 6 subjects from each of two groups. The model estimates a mean for each group and the contrast tests whether the faces–houses activation is stronger in the first group relative to the second group and is an example of a two-sample t-test.

Level 1 model for subject k   Level 2 model for comparing group 1 to group 2

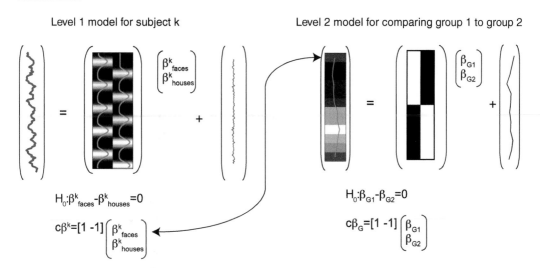

$$H_0: \beta^k_{\text{faces}} - \beta^k_{\text{houses}} = 0$$

$$c\beta^k = [1\ \text{-}1] \begin{pmatrix} \beta^k_{\text{faces}} \\ \beta^k_{\text{houses}} \end{pmatrix}$$

$$H_0: \beta_{G1} - \beta_{G2} = 0$$

$$c\beta_G = [1\ \text{-}1] \begin{pmatrix} \beta_{G1} \\ \beta_{G2} \end{pmatrix}$$

Figure 6.2.   Illustration of the two-stage mixed modeling approach used for fMRI data. The first stage (left) models a single subject's data and the second stage (right) combines the single subject estimates (in this case, six subjects in each of two groups) in a two-sample t-test. The hypothesis of interest is whether activation to visual stimuli of faces versus houses is greater in group 1 versus group 2. The first-stage model estimates the faces–houses ($\beta^k_{\text{faces}} - \beta^k_{\text{houses}}$) for each subject and then this contrast for each of 12 subjects comprises the dependent variable in the group model. The group model design matrix has a regressor for the mean of groups 1 and 2 in the first and second columns, respectively; therefore β_{G1} and β_{G2} represent the means for each group.

See the end of Appendix A for a review of how to set up a wide variety of models using the GLM, including linear regression, one-sample t-tests, two-sample t-tests, paired t-tests, ANOVA, ANCOVA, and repeated measures ANOVA.

The first-level model estimation is carried out as described in the previous chapter. Recall from the previous section that a proper mixed effects model accounts for both within- and between-subject sources of variability. The first-level model supplies us with the within-subject variance estimate and the between-subject variance is estimated in the second-level analysis. There are two different approaches to estimating the between-subject variance used in fMRI software. The most involved approach accounts for the between-subject variance while simultaneously estimating the variance between subjects. This is typically done in an iterative fashion, where the group mean and between-subject variance are alternatively estimated, for details see Worsley et al. (2002) and Woolrich et al. (2004b). In the end, the overall variance for a subject, j, is defined by $\hat{\sigma}^2_{W_j} + \hat{\sigma}^2_B$, where $\hat{\sigma}^2_{W_j}$ is the first-level within-subject variance for subject j and $\hat{\sigma}^2_B$ is the between-subject variance, which is identical for all subjects. The intrasubject variance $\hat{\sigma}^2_{W_j}$ is known from the relatively precise estimates obtained at the first-level model, whereas $\hat{\sigma}^2_B$ must be estimated at the second level, generally on the basis of many fewer observations.

Since each subject's mixed effects variance will likely be different, the weighted linear regression approach described in Appendix A is used, where $(\hat{\sigma}^2_{W_j} + \hat{\sigma}^2_B)^{-1/2}$ is used as a weight for that subject j's data. The essential feature of this approach is that "bad" subjects, those with relatively high $\hat{\sigma}^2_{W_j}$, are down-weighted relative to "good" subjects.

The other approach to estimating the mixed model requires making a simplifying assumption, that the within-subject variances are identical across subjects; this approach allows *ordinary least squares (OLS)* model estimation to be used. The OLS model assumes that all of the $\sigma^2_{W_j}$ are the same, in which case the mixed effects variance is greatly simplified. Let σ^2_W be the common within-subject variance across all subjects, then the mixed effects variance is given by $\sigma^2_W + \sigma^2_B$. Since this value is the same across all subjects, we can just express it as σ^2_{MFX}, a single variance parameter, and OLS will estimate this quantity as the residual variance. In our earlier example of calculating difference in means of the faces–houses contrast, this means that in our group model we are assuming we have a set of observations from a normal distribution with variance σ^2_{MFX}, which simply boils down to carrying out a standard two-sample t-test on the first-level contrast estimates across subjects. In other words, the mean and variance in this model are calculated just as you would in a two-sample t-test. This greatly reduces the computation time for the model estimation, since it is no longer necessary to use iterative methods.

The only downside to this model is that, in practice, the $\sigma^2_{W_j}$ will never be exactly equal over subjects. Perhaps the subject wasn't paying attention or moved a lot in the scanner, increasing the variability of the data compared to other subjects. Also, in many experiments, the number of trials is dependent on the subject's response, and one subject may have very few correct trials and another subject having almost all correct trials. Fortunately, for single-group comparisons, it doesn't make much difference whether OLS or GLS is used at the second level (Mumford & Nichols, 2009). However, if two groups or more are compared, or a second-level regression with a covariate is used, OLS and GLS may give different answers and GLS is to be preferred. See Box 6.1.2 for details on how different software packages fit second-level models.

6.1.3 Fixed effects models

The fixed effects model was described at the beginning of this chapter and only uses the within-subject variance, σ^2_W. The most common use of a fixed effects model is when each subject has multiple runs of data and the runs need to be combined. In this case, the model estimation has three levels: single run, single subject, and group. The single run analysis (first level) is carried out as described in the previous chapter, the single subject analysis (second level) amounts to a weighted average of the first-level effects, and the group analysis (third level) is estimated as discussed in the previous section. Precisely, the second-level analysis combines the per run estimates using a fixed effects model, which is a weighted linear regression with weights simply given by the inverse of the within-run standard deviations that were estimated in

> **Box 6.1.2**   Group modeling in SPM, FSL, & AFNI
>
> SPM, FSL, and AFNI all allow for group modeling but have different assumptions and limitations. SPM does not use first-level variance information in second-level models, and thus only use OLS for simple group models. However, it does allow repeated measures at the group level, for example when you have three or more contrasts per subject that you wish to model together. However, as with first-level fMRI, this correlation is modeled globally (i.e., it is assumed to be the same over all brain voxels).
>
> FSL and AFNI use first-level variance estimates in its second-level model, thus providing estimates using a full mixed effect model. They estimate the random effects variance σ_B^2 at each voxel and so should give the more sensitive estimates when there is heterogeneity in the intrasubject variances $\sigma_{W_j}^2$. However, FSL cannot accommodate repeated measures at the group level, and so all analyses must take the form of one contrast per subject (or, at most, a pair of contrasts per subject, in a paired t-test design). AFNI's 3dMEMA program likewise cannot consider group-level repeated measures, but with the 3dANOVA program, you analyze balanced repeated measures designs.

the first-level analysis, $\frac{1}{\sigma_{W_{r_i}}}$, for each run ($r_i$). Note that in the fixed effects analysis, a new variance term is not estimated and only the within-run variance is used, making inferences only applicable to these runs from this subject. The reason a full mixed effects model cannot be used to combine runs over subjects is because there are not many runs per subject, typically between two and four, making it difficult to reliably estimate the variance since when very few observations are used in the variance estimate, the estimate itself is highly variable and unreliable.

6.2 Mean centering continuous covariates

Although the GLM is capable of estimating a wide range of models from one-sample t-tests to ANCOVA models, setting up these models is sometimes not straightforward. One issue that often arises when setting up models with continuous covariates is that of mean centering the regressors. For example, if you would like to adjust for subject age in the group analysis you can include a variable consisting of the age in years, or you can include a variable that is the age in years minus the mean age of your group. Mean centering (sometimes also called de-meaning) is actually an example of *orthogonalization*, which was described in Section 5.1.3 and is in fact one of the few acceptable uses of orthogonalization. Although mean centering does not change the quality of the fit of the model, it does change the interpretation of some of the parameter estimates, and this impact is important to understand. We start with the model containing only a single group of subjects and then discuss the multiple group problem.

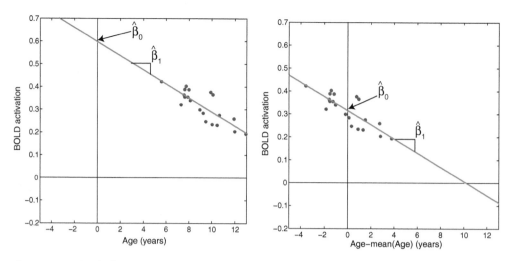

Figure 6.3. Simple linear regression fit before (left) and after (right) mean centering the continuous covariate, Age. In both cases the slope of the line, β_1, is identical, but after age is demeaned, this shifts the data so that the Y intercept of the linear fit is the overall mean of the dependent variable (BOLD activation).

6.2.1 Single group

It is easiest to understand the impact of mean centering a covariate in the case of a simple linear regression. For example, assume the model includes the intercept (column of 1s) as well as an age covariate, $\mathbf{BOLD} = \beta_0 + \beta_1 * \mathbf{Age} + \epsilon$. Without mean-centering age, the interpretation of $\hat{\beta}_0$ is the mean BOLD activation at age 0 (Figure 6.3, left), which is obviously not a very useful interpretation. Instead, if age is mean centered, by replacing each subject's age value with their age minus the mean age over all subjects, the interpretation is more useful. The right side of Figure 6.3 shows the data and model fit when mean-centered age is used and since the data have been shifted to the left, $\hat{\beta}_0$ is now the mean BOLD activation for the subjects in the analysis. Notice that although mean-centering age impacts the estimate of β_0, the estimate for β_1 remains unchanged (the slopes of the fitted regression in the right and left panels of Figure 6.3 match). This is a example of the general fact that when one variable (in this case, the age variable) is orthogonalized with respect to another variable (in this case, the mean BOLD activation), the parameter estimate for the orthogonalized variable does not change while the parameter estimate for the variable orthogonalized against does change.

6.2.2 Multiple groups

In the single group case, it is fairly straightforward to understand why mean centering is appropriate and how it should be carried out, but with two groups the situation is more complicated. Let's start with a simple case, in which there are two groups (males and females) with measures of the BOLD signal corresponding to an emotional face task for each subject. You are interested in whether females would have stronger activation corresponding to the emotional faces than males. The starting point is the two-sample t-test, and you find that the group difference is indeed significant, reflecting the fact that females have more activation than males ($p < .0001$).

Although you have found a difference in BOLD activation according to gender with the two-sample t-test, it may be the case that depression level, another measure you have collected on all subjects, explains the differences in BOLD activation better than gender. In other words, it could simply be the case that males are less depressed than females, and depression differences, not gender differences, describe the variability in the BOLD activation corresponding to emotional faces. To test whether this is the case, you would add depression as a regressor to the two-sample t-test model as shown in the left panel of Figure 6.4. Your primary interest is in the group effect and whether it remains when depression level is added to the model, so you test the contrast $c_1 = [1 \ -1 \ 0]$ and find that after adjusting for depression levels across subjects there is no longer a gender difference in the BOLD response to emotional faces ($p = .56$). In addition, a contrast for the depression effect ($c_2 = [0 \ 0 \ 1]$) is significant with $p < .0001$. In other words, the differences in BOLD activation are not due to gender, but are best explained by a subject's depression level. In this case, mean centering has no impact on the contrast that tests for the group difference (c_2) because the model is fitting two lines, one for each gender, with different intercepts

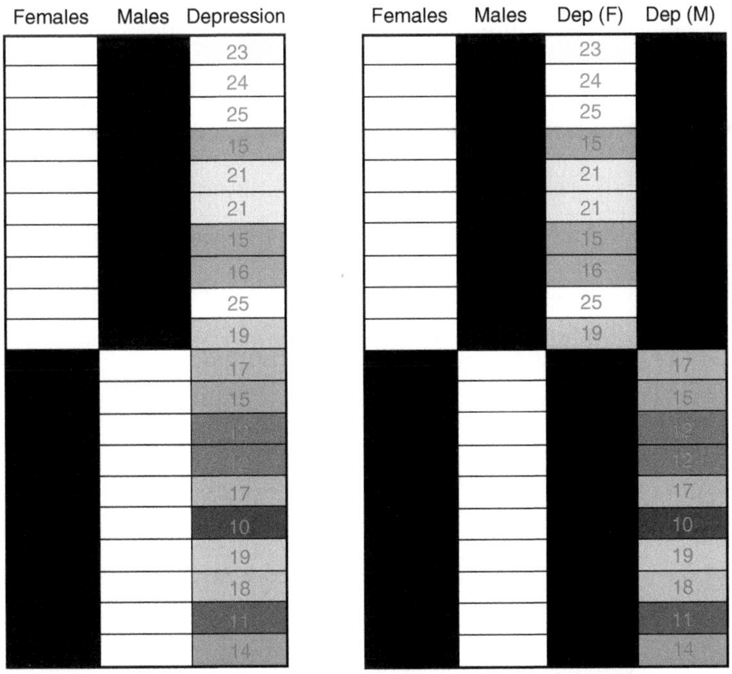

Figure 6.4.   Design matrices when adding depression level to a two sample t-test. The left panel demonstrates the model with only a main effect for depression, whereas the right panel illustrates the model with an gender/depression interaction. The numbers in red correspond to the depression scores for the subjects (without mean centering).

and matching slopes. The lines are parallel, and so the difference in BOLD activation for any level of depression is constant.

A common step after this is to test for a gender/depression interaction, which tests whether males and females exhibit different relationships between their BOLD activations and depression levels. For example, it may be that as depression level increases, the increase in BOLD activation is faster for females than males. The model with no mean centering is shown in the right panel of Figure 6.4. Mean centering in this model is more confusing, since one could either subtract the overall mean depression or the mean depression within each gender group, since each group has a separate depression regressor. In models that include interaction effects, we typically ignore the main effects and focus first on whether or not the interaction itself ($c = [0\ 0\ 1\ -1]$) is significant (see Box 6.2.2). However, sometimes we may wish to look at the gender difference at a specific depression level, corresponding to the contrast $c_3 = [1\ -1\ 0\ 0]$, and this is where mean centering is important. If one were to mean center using the mean depression score across all subjects, then the contrast c_3 would correspond to the difference in BOLD according to gender for the average depression level. On the other hand, if the depression score is mean centered within each gender group, the interpretation of c_3 is the gender difference for the average depression level *not* adjusted for gender-specific differences in depression. In this case, c_3 will often be significant and will be misinterpreted as a difference in gender adjusted for depression level, when in fact such mean centering prevents any adjustment between genders by depression level! Because of this, mean centering within group should *never* be done. It not only confuses the interpretation of c_3 but also of the model in general.

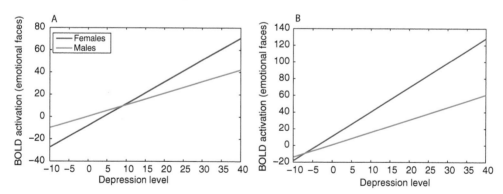

Figure 6.5.   Two examples of significant gender/depression interactions. Panel A shows a model fit where the cross occurs at a depression level around 10, whereas panel B shows an example where the lines cross outside of the possible values of depression (scores range between 0 and 40 for this measure). In both cases, the change in BOLD activation as depression increases is stronger for females than males (the female slope is larger). Since in panel B the lines cross outside of the range, we can also conclude that within reasonable limits, the BOLD activation is stronger for females than males. For panel A, the BOLD activation is stronger for females for depression levels greater than 10, whereas males have stronger BOLD activation for depression levels less than 10.

Box 6.2.2 Understanding models with significant interactions

When you model an interaction between a categorical covariate and a continuous covariate, as shown in the right panel of Figure 6.4, you are basically fitting a simple linear regression for males and females separately, allowing both the intercepts and linear trend associated with depression to vary by gender group. If the interaction is significant, it means that the slopes of these lines differ and that the lines will cross for some value of depression. Figure 6.5 shows two examples of model fits when there was a significant gender/depression interaction in the model. When looking at these fitted models, it is easy to see that what is perhaps the most interesting is where the lines cross and how they behave before and after this crossing point. If the cross occurs at a depression level that is meaningful, such as in panel A, then this tells us that below this depression level females have lower BOLD activation than males and above this depression level females have higher BOLD activations. We often call this a crossover interaction because the response crosses over at meaningful values of the variable. On the other hand, in panel B the lines would cross for a negative value of depression level, which does not actually occur in the data. In this case, it is interesting that females always have stronger activation than males and that their change in BOLD activation as depression increases is much stronger than the change in male BOLD activation. Note that finding this crossing point requires using all four parameter estimates from the model (occurs when depression is $(\beta_2 - \beta_1)/(\beta_3 - \beta_4)$), which is often difficult to do in an imaging analysis unless you are focusing on a single region of interest. Typically in a whole brain analysis the focus is on whether or not the slope for males is greater or less than the slope for females (so $c = [0\ 0\ 1\ -1]$ or $c = [0\ 0\ -1\ 1]$).

The important thing to note is that the main effect of group reflects the difference in activation at the average depression level across subjects, and does not tell us where the lines cross. This is the reason why we generally do not interpret main effects when they occur in the context of interactions, because they can be misleading.

## 7

Statistical inference on images

The goal of statistical inference is to make decisions based on our data, while accounting for uncertainty due to noise in the data. From a broad perspective, statistical inference on fMRI data is no different from traditional data analysis on, say, a response time dataset. Inference for fMRI is challenging, however, because of the massive nature of the datasets and their spatial form. Thus, we need to define precisely what are the features of the images that we want to make inference on, and we have to account for the multiplicity in searching over the brain for an effect.

We begin with a brief review of traditional univariate statistical inference and then discuss the different features in images we can make inference on and finally cover the very important issue of multiple testing.

7.1 Basics of statistical inference

We will first briefly review the concepts of classical hypothesis testing, which is the main approach used for statistical inference in fMRI analysis. A *null hypothesis H_0* is an assertion about a parameter, some feature of the population from which we're sampling. H_0 is the default case, typically that of "no effect," and the *alternative hypothesis H_1* corresponds to the scientific hypothesis of interest. A *test statistic T* is a function of the data that summarizes the evidence against the null hypothesis. We write T for the yet-to-be-observed (random valued) test statistic, and t for a particular observed value of T. (Note here T stands for a generic *Test* statistic, not t-test.) While there are many different possible types of test statistics with different units and interpretations (e.g., t-tests, F-tests, χ^2-tests), the *P-value* expresses the evidence against H_0 for any type of T: The P-value is $P(T \geq t | H_0)$, the chance under the null hypothesis of observing a test statistic as large or larger than actually observed. (Tests for decreases in T or two-sided changes, i.e., either positive or negative, are possible by redefining T.)

It is useful to dispense with two frequent misunderstandings about P-values. First, and crucially, the P-value *is not* the probability that the null is true given the data, $P(H_0|T)$. To determine this quantity, we must use Bayesian computations that are not part of Classical hypothesis testing (see Box 7.1). Roughly, the P-value expresses the surprise of observing the data if the null hypothesis was actually true. Second, a P-value can only be used to refute H_0 and doesn't provide evidence for the truth of H_0. The reason for this is that the P-value computation begins by assuming that the null hypothesis is true, and thus a P-value cannot be used to deduce that H_0 is true.

When P-values are used to decide whether to reject H_0 or not, there are two different types of errors that one can make, and we can quantify the likelihood of each. Rejecting H_0 when there is no effect is a Type I or false positive error. The desired tolerance of the chance of a false positive is the *Type I error level*, denoted α. Failing to reject H_0 when there truly is an effect is a Type II or false negative error. The chance that a testing procedure correctly rejects H_0 when there is a true effect is the *power* of the procedure (which is one minus the Type II error rate). Power varies as a function of the size of the true effect, the efficiency of the statistical procedure, and the sample size. This implies that a sample size that is sufficient to detect an effect in one study (which has a relatively large effect magnitude using a sensitive statistical test) may not be sufficient to find an effect in other studies where the true effect is smaller or the test is less sensitive. In Section 7.6 we consider power calculations in detail.

For any testing procedure used to make "Reject"/"Don't Reject" decisions, based either on T or on P, there are several ways to describe the performance of the test. A test is said to be *valid* if the chance of a Type I error is less than or equal to α; if this chance exceeds α, we say the test is *invalid* or *anticonservative*. A test is *exact* if the chance of a Type I error is precisely α, while if this probability is strictly less than α we say the test is *conservative*. In this terminology, we always seek to use valid tests, and among valid tests we seek those with the greatest power.

Box 7.1 Bayesian statistics and inference

Bayesian methods are growing in popularity, as they provide a means to express prior knowledge before we see the data. Thomas Bayes (1702–61) is remembered for the following theorem:

$$P(A|B) = \frac{P(B|A)P(A)}{P(B)}$$

which says the chance of random event A occurring assuming or *given* that B occurs, can be computed from an expression involving the reverse statement, the chance of B given A. This expression gives a formal mechanism for combining prior information with information in the data. In the context of the GLM with data y and parameters β, it allows us to write $f(\beta|y) \propto f(y|\beta)f(\beta)$, where $f(\beta)$ is the *prior* density, our beliefs about the parameters before we see the data (e.g., that BOLD percent changes generally range from -5% to $+5\%$), $f(y|\beta)$ is the traditional likelihood of the data given parameters, and $f(\beta|y)$ is the posterior, the distribution of the parameter after we observe the data. Crucially, it allows us to make probabilistic statements on the unknown parameter β, whereas classical (or *frequentist*) statistics assumes β is fixed and has no random variation. Bayesian inference is based entirely on the posterior: The posterior mean provides a point estimate, and the posterior standard deviation provides the equivalent of a standard error.

There are fundamental differences between the classical and Bayesian approaches. A classical method couches inference relative to infinite theoretical replications of your experiment: A 95% confidence interval means that if you were to repeat your experiment over and over, 19 out of 20 times (on average) the interval produced will cover the fixed, true, but unobservable parameter. The randomness of the data over hypothetical experimental replications drives frequentist inference. The Bayesian method casts inference based on belief about the *random* unobservable parameter: The prior expresses belief about the parameter before seeing the data, the posterior expresses belief about the parameter after seeing the data. There is no reference to infinite replications of your experiment, as the data are fixed (not random).

A true Bayesian thinks a classical statistician is absurd for referencing imaginary experiments that are never conducted. A true classical statistician thinks a Bayesian is irrational because different scientists (with different priors) could analyze the same data and come to different conclusions. Fortunately, in many settings the Bayesian and classical methods give similar answers, because with more and more data the influence of the prior diminishes and the posterior looks like the classical likelihood function.

7.2 Features of interest in images

For an image composed of V voxels, it might seem that there is only one way to decide where there is a signal, by testing each and every voxel individually. This approach is referred to as 'voxel-level' inference. Alternatively, we can take into account the spatial information available in the images, by finding connected clusters of activated voxels and testing the significance of each cluster, which is referred to as 'cluster-level' inference. (See Figure 7.1.) Finally, we might sometimes simply want to ask 'is there any significant activation anywhere?' which is referred to as a 'set-level' inference. First, we discuss what it means to have a significant voxel-level or cluster-level result,

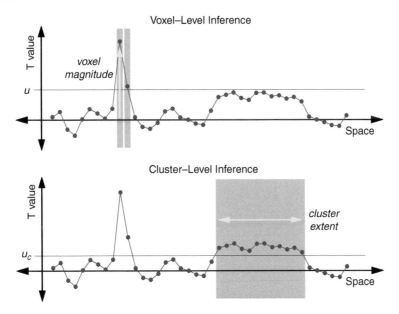

Figure 7.1.   Illustration of voxel-level versus cluster-level inference. Both axes show the same one-dimensional section of a statistic image. In the top, voxel-level inference finds two voxels above a significance threshold, and thus both voxels are individually marked as significant. In the bottom, a cluster-forming threshold defines clusters, and cluster-wise inference finds a single cluster of 12 voxels significant; none of the 12 voxels are individually significant, but together they comprise a significant cluster.

and then how we actually compute significance (P-values) accounting for the search over the brain.

7.2.1 Voxel-level inference

In an image of test statistics, each voxel's value measures the evidence against the null hypothesis at that location. The most spatially specific inference that we can make is to determine whether there is a significant effect at each individual voxel. We do this by examining whether the statistic at each voxel exceeds a threshold u; if it does, then we mark that voxel as being "significant" (i.e., we reject the null hypothesis at that voxel). Such voxel-by-voxel inferences allow us to make very specific inferences if the threshold is chosen properly; in Section 7.3 we discuss how the threshold is chosen.

7.2.2 Cluster-level inference

Voxel-level inferences make no use of any spatial information in the image, such as the fact that activated voxels might be clustered together in space. However, we generally expect that the signals in fMRI will be spatially extended. One reason is that the brain regions that are activated in fMRI are often much larger than the size of a single voxel. The second reason is that fMRI data are often spatially smoothed and then oversampled to small (e.g., 2 mm^3) voxels during spatial normalization, which results in a spreading of the signal across many voxels in the image.

To take advantage of this knowledge about the spatial structure of fMRI signals, it is most common to make inferences about clusters of activated voxels rather than about individual voxels, which is referred to as *cluster-level inference*. The most common approach to cluster-level inference involves a two-step procedure. First, a primary threshold (known as a *cluster-forming threshold*) u_c is applied to a statistic image, and the groups of contiguous voxels above u_c are defined as 'clusters'. What exactly constitutes 'contiguous' depends on the definition of a neighborhood. For example, in 2D, we certainly would consider two suprathreshold voxels connected if they share an edge (4-connectivity), but might also consider them connected if they share a corner (8-connectivity). In 3D, the choices are 6-connectivity (only faces), 18-connectivity (also edges) or 26-connectivity (also corners).[1] Second, the significance of each cluster is determined by measuring its size (in voxels) and comparing this to a critical cluster size threshold k. Methods for choosing this threshold k are discussed below in Section 7.3.

Cluster size inference is generally more sensitive than voxel-level inference for standard MRI data (Friston et al., 1996a). In rough terms, cluster size inference should be better at detecting a signal when that signal is larger in scale than the smoothness of the noise. To see this, consider an example where our fMRI noise has smoothness of 10 mm FWHM and the true effects are also 10 mm in scale. In this instance, the true signal clusters will be similar in size to noise-only clusters, and it will be difficult for cluster-level inference to detect the signal. In contrast, if the scale of the effect is larger than 10 mm, cluster-level inference should detect the effects more often than voxel-level inference. Assigning signifiance to clusters based on their extent ignores the statistic values within a cluster. It would seem that using such intensity information would improve the sensitivity of cluster inference, and indeed some authors have found this result. Poline & Mazoyer (1993) proposed inference using the minimum of the cluster size P-value and cluster peak P-value, and Bullmore et al. (1999) suggested *cluster mass* inference based on the sum of all voxel-level statistic values in a cluster. For the mass statistic in particular, Hayasaka & Nichols (2004) found that it has equal or greater power than the size statistic.

There are two drawbacks to cluster-level inference: The arbitrary cluster-forming threshold and the lack of spatial specificity. The cluster-forming threshold u_c can be set to any value in principle, though if set too low, focal signal may be lost in the gigantic clusters that are formed, and if set too high it may exclude voxels with weak signal intensity (see Figure 7.2). Also, random field theory results break down for thresholds more generous than $\alpha = 0.01$ (see Section 7.3.1). Most troubling, if one

---

[1] The SPM software uses 18-connectivity while the FSL uses 26-connectivity; in practice you find very similar clusters with either connectivity unless the data has very low smoothness.

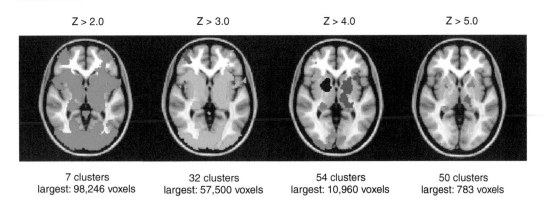

| Z > 2.0 | Z > 3.0 | Z > 4.0 | Z > 5.0 |

| 7 clusters | 32 clusters | 54 clusters | 50 clusters |
| largest: 98,246 voxels | largest: 57,500 voxels | largest: 10,960 voxels | largest: 783 voxels |

Figure 7.2.   Effects of cluster-forming threshold on cluster size. The same data were thresholded using increasing cluster-size thresholds; the resulting clusters are randomly color-coded to show which voxels belong to each cluster. At the lowest threshold, there is one large cluster that encompasses much of the brain, whereas higher thresholds break up this cluster, at the expense of excluding many regions that do not survive the higher threshold.

adjusts u_c up or down just slightly, some clusters may merge or split, and significant clusters disappear. In practice, most users take u_c to correspond to either $\alpha = 0.01$ or $\alpha = 0.001$ (FSL users must set a statistic value threshold rather than a P-value, usually $z = 2.3$ or 3.1).

Cluster inference's greater power comes at the expense of spatial specificity, or precision. When a 1,000 voxel cluster is marked as statistically significant, we cannot point to a single voxel in the cluster and say "The signal is here." All we can conclude is that one or more voxels within that cluster have evidence against the null. This isn't a problem, though, when cluster sizes are small. If you get a cluster that covers half the brain, however, this can be quite unsatisfying. The only remedy is to resort to raising u_c to get smaller clusters, but this further compounds the multiple testing problem because one is searching across multiple thresholds.

A recently developed method attempts to address these two problems. Threshold Free Cluster Enhancement (TFCE) (Smith & Nichols, 2009) uses all possible u_c, and then integrates over u_c to provide a voxel-level map that indicates cluster-level significance. By eliminating one parameter it does introduce two new parameters, specifically how to weight u_c versus cluster size, but these are set to fixed values inspired by theory and empirical simulations. While not an established approach, it has shown promise as a sensitive approach to cluster-level inference that removes the dependence on the cluster-forming threshold.

7.2.3 Set-level inference

Although rare, there may be some cases when one simply wants to know if there is any significant activation for a particular contrast, with no concern for where the activation is. In SPM, there is an inference method known as *set-level inference* that

---

Box 7.2.3 Inference on location vs. inference on magnitude

When we apply a threshold to a statistic image and search the brain for activations, the end result is an inference on location. We answer the question: "*Where* in the brain is there a response to my experiment?" Once a significant region is identified as active, one would like to characterize the nature of the effect, in particular the effect magnitude. However, due to a problem of *circularity* (discussed in greater detail in Chapter 10; see Box 10.4.2), we cannot subsequently answer the question of *how large* the identified effect is. The reason is that of all the possible true positive voxels we will detect, we are more likely to find the voxels that are randomly higher than the true effect and will miss those that are randomly smaller. In genetics this is known as the "winner's curse," as the first group to find a gene will often report an effect size that is greater than any subsequent replication.

At the present time, there is no way to correct for the bias in effect sizes found by searching the brain for activations. One simply must recognize that effect size bias is present and note this when discussing the result. If unbiased effect size estimates are required, one must sacrifice inference on location and instead assume a fixed and known location for the effect. Specifically, one must use a priori specified regions of interest (ROIs) and average the data within those regions. For more on the topic of circularity, see Kriegeskorte et al. (2009).

---

is an overall test of whether there exists any significant signals anywhere in the brain. The test statistic is the number of clusters for an arbitrary cluster defining threshold u_c that are larger than an arbitrary cluster size threshold k. A significant set-level P-value indicates that there are an unusually large number of clusters present, but it doesn't indicate *which* clusters are significant. For this reason it is referred to an *omnibus* test and has no localizing power whatsoever.

7.3 The multiple testing problem and solutions

As previously reviewed, classical statistical methods provide a straightforward means to control the level of false positive risk through appropriate selection of α. However, this guarantee is a made only on a test-by-test basis. If a statistic image has 100,000 voxels, and we declare all voxels with $P < 0.05$ to be "significant," then on average 5% of the 100,000 voxels – 5,000 voxels – will be false positives! This problem is referred to as the *multiple testing problem* and is a critical issue for fMRI analysis.

Standard hypothesis tests are designed only to control the 'per comparison rate' and are not meant to be used repetitively for a set of related tests. To account for the multiplicity, we have to measure false positive risk over an entire image. We define, in turn, two measures of false positive risk – the familywise error rate and the false discovery rate.

7.3.1 Familywise error rate

The most common measure of Type I error over multiple tests is the 'familywise error rate', abbreviated FWER or FWE. FWE is the chance of one or more false positives anywhere in the image. When we use a valid procedure with $\alpha_{FWE} = 0.05$, there is at most a 5% chance of *any* false positives anywhere in the map. Equivalently, after thresholding with a valid $\alpha_{FWE} = 0.05$ threshold, we have 95% confidence that there are no false positive voxels (or clusters) in the thresholded map. For a particular voxel (or cluster), we can refer to its "corrected FWE *P*-value" or just "corrected *P*-value," which is the smallest α_{FWE} that allows detection of that voxel (or cluster).

Several procedures that can provide valid corrected P-values for fMRI data are available.

7.3.1.1 Bonferroni correction

Perhaps the most widely known method for controlling FWE is the 'Bonferroni correction.' By using a threshold of $\alpha = \alpha_{FWE}/V$, where V is the number of tests, we will have a valid FWE procedure for any type of data. However, even though it will control FWE for any dataset, the Bonferroni procedure becomes conservative when there is strong correlation between tests. Because of the smoothness of fMRI data, Bonferroni corrections are usually very strongly conservative. Instead, we need a method that accounts for the spatial dependence between voxels. The two main methods that do this are random field theory (RFT) and permutation methods.

7.3.1.2 Random field theory

Random field theory uses an elegant mathematical theory on the topology of thresholded images. The details of this method require mathematics beyond the scope of this book, but an approachable overview can be found in Nichols & Hayasaka (2003); treatments with more mathematical detail can be found in Cao & Worsley (2001) and Adler & Taylor (2007).

A crucial aspect of RFT is how it accounts for the degree of smoothness in the data. Smoothness is measured by $FWHM = [FWHM_x, FWHM_y, FWHM_z]$. This smoothness is *not* the size of the Gaussian smoothing kernel applied to the data, but rather the intrinsic smoothness of the data. That is, even before any smoothing, there is some spatial correlation present in all imaging data, and the RFT smoothness parameter relates to the combination of the intrinsic and applied smoothing.

The definition of RFT's FWHM is somewhat convoluted: It is the size of a Gaussian kernel that, when applied to spatially independent "white noise" data, induces the degree of smoothness present in the noise of the data at hand. See previous citations for a more precise definition in terms of the variability of the partial derivatives of the noise.

A related concept is 'RESEL' or RESolution ELement, a virtual voxel of size $\text{FWHM}_x \times \text{FWHM}_y \times \text{FWHM}_z$. The analysis volume expressed in units of RESELs is denoted R, the RESEL count.

We present one formula to gain intuition on how RFT results work, the expression for the corrected P-value for a voxel value t in a three-dimensional Gaussian statistic image

$$P_{\text{FWE}}^{\text{vox}}(t) \approx R \times \frac{(4\ln(2))^{3/2}}{(2\pi)^2} e^{-t^2/2}(t^2 - 1) \tag{7.1}$$

where $R = V/(\text{FWHM}_x\text{FWHM}_y\text{FWHM}_z)$ is the RESEL count for the image. This demonstrates the essential role of the RESEL count and shows that, for a given statistic value t and search volume V, as the product of FWHM's increase, the RESEL count decreases and so does the corrected P-value, producing increased significance. The intuition is that greater smoothness means there is a less severe multiple testing problem, and a less stringent correction is necessary. Conversely, as the search volume in RESELs grows, so does the corrected P-value, producing decreased significance for the same statistical value. This should also make sense, as the larger the search volume, the more severe the multiple testing problem.

These observations illustrate how RFT inference adapts to the smoothness in the data, and how the RESEL count is related to the number of 'independent observations' in the image. This loose interpretation, however, is far as it goes, and RFT should never be misunderstood to be equivalent to a 'RESEL-based Bonferroni correction'. This is not the case, and there is no equivalent voxel count that you can feed into Bonferroni correction that will match RFT inferences (Nichols & Hayasaka, 2003).

RFT can also be used to obtain P-values for the clusters based on cluster-size (Friston et al., 1994b). Again, the details are mathematically involved, but Gaussian random field theory provides results for the expected size and number of clusters, and these results adapt to the smoothness of the search volume. RFT P-values have also been developed for the alternate cluster statistics mentioned earlier, combined cluster size and peak height (Poline & Mazoyer, 1993) and cluster mass (Zhang et al., 2009).

Limitations of RFT. Even though RFT methods form the core of fMRI inference, they have a number of shortcomings. First, they require a multitude of distributional assumptions and approximations. In particular, they require that the random field be sufficiently smooth, which practically means that one needs to smooth the data with a Gaussian filter whose FWHM is at least twice the voxel dimensions. In fact, the RFT methods are overly conservative for smoothness less than three- to four-voxel FWHM (Nichols & Hayasaka, 2003; Hayasaka & Nichols, 2003). In addition,

RFT methods are overly conservative for sample sizes less than about 20 (Nichols & Hayasaka, 2003; Hayasaka & Nichols, 2003).

7.3.1.3 Parametric simulations

Another approach to voxel-level and cluster-level inference is Monte Carlo simulation, from which we can find a threshold that controls the FWE. For example, Forman et al. (1995) proposed a Monte Carlo cluster-level inference method. Gaussian data are simulated and smoothed based on the estimated smoothness of the real data, creating surrogate statistic images under the null hypothesis. These surrogate images are thresholded, and an empirical cluster size distribution is derived. These methods have an underlying model that is similar to RFT's model (i.e., smooth Gaussian data), but they do not rely on an asymptotic or approximate results. They are, however, much more computationally intensive than RFT.

This method is implemented in AFNI's alphasim program. Users of this approach must take care that the smoothness parameter, which, as in RFT, is not the size of the applied smoothing kernel but the estimated intrinsic smoothness of the data. In addition, the analysis mask used for the simulation must be exactly the same as the mask used for analysis of the real data.

7.3.1.4 Nonparametric approaches

Instead of making parametric assumptions about the data to approximate P-values, an alternative approach is to use the data themselves to obtain empirical null distributions of the test statistic of interest. The two most widely used resampling methods are permutation tests and the bootstrap. While the bootstrap is perhaps better known, it is an asymptotic method (meaning that it is only provably correct in the large-sample limit), and in particular has been shown to have poor performance for estimating FWE-corrected P-values (Troendle et al., 2004). In contrast the permutation test, which has exact control of false positive risk, is a useful alternative to RFT methods for small samples.

A permutation test is easy to understand when comparing two groups. Considering just a single voxel, suppose you have two groups of ten subjects, high performers (H) and low performers (L), each of whose BOLD response data you wish to compare. Under the null hypothesis of no group difference, the group labels are arbitrary, and one could randomly select ten subjects to be the H group, reanalyze the data, and expect similar results. This is the principle of the permutation test: repeatedly shuffling the assignment of experimental labels to the data, and analyzing the data for each shuffle to create a distribution of statistic values that would be expected under the null hypothesis. Just as a parametric P-value is found by integrating the tails of the null distribution that are more extreme than the actual data observed, the nonparametric permutation P-value is the proportion of the permuted statistic values that are as or more extreme than the value that was actually observed. See Figure 7.3 for an illustration of this example with three subjects per group.

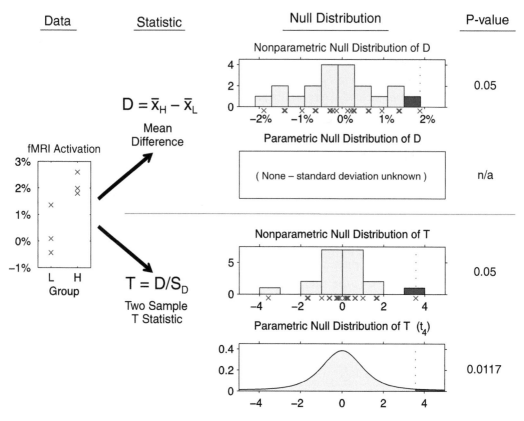

Figure 7.3.   Illustration of parametric and nonparametric inference at the group level, comparing two groups of three subjects. Parametric methods use assumptions about the data to find the null distribution of the test statistic. Nonparametric methods use the data itself to find the null distribution, allowing the consideration of nonstandard test statistics. Under the null hypothesis the group labels are irrelevant, and thus we can reanalyze the data over and over with different permutations of the labels. Here, there are 20 possible ways to assign three subjects to the Low-performers group (and the other three must be high performers), and thus the permutation distribution consists of 20 test statistic values. With either parametric or nonparametric methods, the P-value is the proportion of the null distribution as large or larger than the statistic actually observed. However, there is no parametric test for the difference, as the standard deviation (S_D) is unknown.

For a single subject's fMRI data, the permutation test is difficult to apply. Drift and temporal autocorrelation make the timeseries autocorrelated and thus not "exchangeable" under the null hypothesis (since randomly reordering the data points would disrupt the temporal autocorrelation). Even though there are methods to decorrelate the data (Bullmore et al., 2001) as part of the permutation procedure, such *semiparametric* methods are very computationally demanding and depend on accurate modelling of the correlation.

At the group level, on the other hand, the permutation approach is easy to apply (this correction is implemented in the *randomise* tool in FSL and in the *SnPM* toolbox for SPM). Each subject is analyzed with a standard GLM model, and for each contrast of interest, an effect image (a Contrast of Parameter Estimates or COPE image in FSL; a con image in SPM) is created. If there is just a single group of subjects, it might seem that a permutation test is impossible, as there are no group labels to permute. If we instead assume that the COPE images have a symmetric distribution (about zero under H_0), a permutation test can be made by randomly multiplying each subject's COPE by 1 or -1. The assumption of symmetry is much weaker than a Gaussian assumption and can be justified by the first-level errors having a symmetric distribution.

So far, we have discussed the use of permutation tests to obtain null distributions at each voxel, but this does not solve the multiple testing problem. Importantly, permutation can also be used to obtain FWE-corrected P-values. An FWE-corrected P-value is found by comparing a particular statistic value to the distribution of the maximal statistic across the whole image. In the previous High and Low performers example, this means that for each random labeling of Hs and Ls, the entire brain volume is analyzed, and the maximum statistic value across the whole brain is noted. In the case of voxel-level inference, this is the largest intensity in the statistic image, whereas for cluster-level inference, this is the size of the largest cluster in the image. With repeated permutation a distribution of the maximum statistic is constructed, and the FWE corrected P-value is the proportion of maxima in the permutation distribution that is as large or larger than the observed statistic value.

The primary drawback of permutation methods is that they are computationally intensive. Whereas RFT computations take seconds at most, a typical permutation analysis can take anywhere from 10 minutes to an hour on modern computing hardware. However, given the great amount of time spent to perform other aspects of fMRI processing, this seems like a relatively small price to pay for the accuracy that comes from using permutation tests. In general, when FWE-corrected results are desired, we recommend the use of permutation tests for all inferences on group fMRI data.

7.3.2 False discovery rate

While FWE-corrected voxel-level tests were the first methods available for neuroimaging, practitioners often found the procedures to be quite insensitive, leaving them with no results that survived correction. While sometimes FWE inferences are conservative due to inaccurate RFT methods, even with exact permutation FWE methods, many experiments will produce no positive results (especially with small sample sizes). A more lenient alternative to FWE correction is the false discovery rate (Benjamini & Hochberg, 1995; Genovese et al., 2002). The false discovery proportion (FDP) is the fraction of detected voxels (or clusters) that are false positives (defined as 0 if there are no detected voxels). FDP is unobservable, but FDR procedures guarantee that the average FDP is controlled. Put another way, where a level 0.05 FWE procedure is correct 95% of the time – no more than 5% of experiments

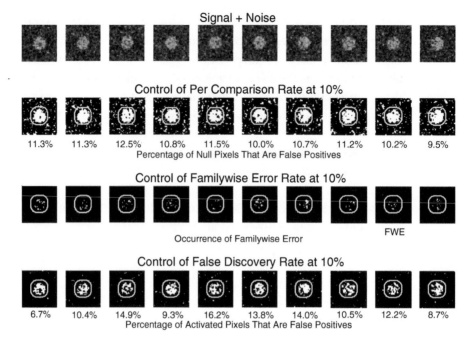

Figure 7.4.   Illustration of three different multiple comparison procedures. Each column corresponds to a different realization of signal plus noise, as illustrated in the simulated data in the top row, and can be thought of as your next ten experiments. The top row shows the statistic image without any thresholding. The second row illustrates the control of the per comparison rate at 10%, that is, no special account of multiplicity. The third row shows control of the familywise error rate at 10%, say with RFT or Bonferroni. The bottom row shows control of the false discovery rate. With no adjustment for multiple testing (second row) there is excellent sensitivity, but very poor specificity – there are false positives everywhere. Controlling FWE (third row) gives excellent specificity – only 1 out of 10 experiments have *any* false positives– but poor sensitivity. Controlling FDR (bottom row) is a compromise between no correction and FWE correction, giving greater sensitivity at the expense of some false positives, even though it is still controlled as a fraction of all voxels detected. Note that, just as the empirical per comparison error rate for each experiment is never exactly 10%, likewise the empirical false discovery rate is never exactly 10%; in both instances, we're guaranteed only that, in the long run, the average rate will not exceed 10%. The yellow circle in each image indicates the region with signal. In the first row, the numbers below each image indicate the proportion of noise (no-signal) voxels falsely detected. In the middle row, the "FWE" label indicates the realization with one or more false positives. And in the bottom row the numbers indicate the proportion of detected voxels that are false positives, the false discovery proportion.

examined can have *any* false positives – a level 0.05 FDR procedure produces results that are 95% correct – in the long run the average FDP will be no more than 5%. (See Figure 7.4.)

FDR's greater sensitivity comes at the cost of greater false positive risk. That risk is still measured in an objective way that accounts for features of the data, which is in contrast to, say, an uncorrected $\alpha = 0.001$ threshold, which will give varying false positive risk depending on smoothness and the size of the search region. Standard

FDR, as applied voxel-level, lacks any kind of spatial specificity, similar to cluster inference. Given a map of FDR-significant voxels, one cannot point to a single voxel and conclude that it is significant. One can only assert that, on average, no more than 5% (or the FDR level used) of the voxels present are false positives. Even if some significant voxels form a large cluster, and others are scattered as tiny clusters, voxel-level FDR has no spatial aspect and does not factor cluster size into significance.

This lack of spatial precision has led some to criticise FDR, with Chumbley & Friston (2009) even recommending that voxel-level FDR should not be used at all. They propose, instead, that FDR should be applied in a cluster-level fashion. On balance, both voxel-level and cluster-level FDR are reasonable procedures, and each needs to be interpreted with care, accounting for the presence of false positives in the map of significant voxels or clusters.

7.3.3 Inference example

To illustrate these inference methods just discussed, we consider data from a gambling task (Tom et al., 2007); these data are available from the book Web site. In this experiment, 16 subjects were offered 50/50 gambles where the size of the potential gain and loss varied parametrically from trial to trial. Here we just consider the negative parametric effect of potential loss on BOLD response (which identifies regions whose activity goes down as the size of the potential loss goes up). Using a cluster-forming threshold of $Z = 2.3$, 154 clusters were found (Figure 7.5a). Based on the search volume and estimated smoothness, RFT finds 5% FWE critical cluster size threshold to be 570 voxels, and only four clusters are larger (Figure 7.5b and Table 7.1).

Note the difficulty in visualizing 3D clusters with orthogonal slices. In Figure 7.5b, in the coronal (middle) slice, there appears to be perhaps six or more separate clusters, yet in fact there are only three clusters shown this panel. Contiguity of clusters is measured in 3D and is very difficult to gauge visually from 2-D slices.

Another challenge arises with large clusters, such as the first cluster in Table 7.1 and as seen in the lower portions of the sagittal and coronal (left and middle) slices. This cluster covers a number of anatomical regions, yet calling this cluster significant only tells us there is some signal somewhere in these 6,041 voxels. If we had known this would be a problem a prori, we could have used voxel-level inference instead to improve spatial specificity. For this data, though, no voxels are found significant with either FWE or FDR (max voxel $Z = 4.00$ has $P_{\text{FWE}}^{\text{vox}} = 1.0$, $P_{\text{FDR}}^{\text{vox}} = 0.1251$). This is typical of cluster inference greater sensitivity over voxel-level inference.

7.4 Combining inferences: masking and conjunctions

A single fMRI experiment will usually produce a number of different contrasts, and fully understanding the outcome of the study may require combining the statistic

(a) All clusters created with Z=2.3 cluster-forming threshold

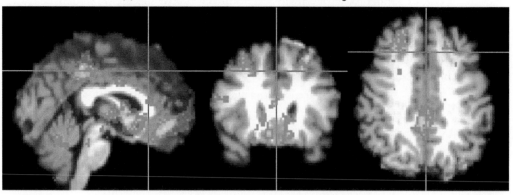

(b) Clusters surviving 5% FWE threshold

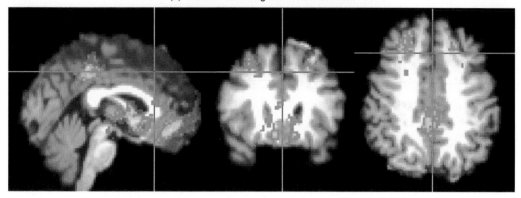

Figure 7.5.   Thresholded maps from the gambling experiment, parametric effect of the size of potential loss on BOLD response. Top (a) shows clusters created with $Z = 2.3$ cluster-forming threshold and no cluster-size threshold, while bottom (b) shows the 3 clusters that survive a critical cluster size threshold of 570 voxels.

Table 7.1.   Significant clusters from the gambling experiment.

Region	Cluster Size (voxels)	Corrected P-value $p_{\text{FWE}}^{\text{clus}}$	X	Y	Z
Striatum, ventromedial prefrontal cortex, ventral anterior cingulate cortex, medial orbitofrontal cortex	6,041	<0.0001	0	4	−4
Right superior frontal gyrus	1,102	0.0010	22	42	38
Posterior cingulate	901	0.0040	4	−38	40
Left superior frontal gyrus	738	0.0133	−30	24	54

Notes: Search volume: 236,516 $2 \times 2 \times 2$ mm^3 voxels, 1.89 liters, 1,719.1 RESELs, FWHM 5.1 mm
Cluster forming threshold $Z = 2.3$, 0.05 FWE cluster size threshold $k = 570$.
[a]Of the 154 clusters found (see Figure 7.5) with a cluster-forming threshold of $Z = 2.3$, only the four listed here are FWE significant at 0.05. X, Y, Z coordinates listed are the location of the peak Z value in each cluster.

images in different ways. To make these issues concrete, consider a 2×2 factorial design, where there are two factors with two levels each. Henson et al. (2002) uses such a design for a face recognition and implicit memory. That study has two factors, "Fame" indicating whether a presented face is famous or nonfamous and "Repetition" indicating whether this is the first or second presentation of a face (each face was presented exactly twice). Among the contrasts of interest are: $c_{Famous>Nonfamous}$, the positive effect of famousness, averaged over both presentations; $c_{Famous:Rep1>Nonfamous:Rep1}$, the famousness effect on the first presentation; $c_{Famous:Rep2>Nonfamous:Rep2}$, the famousness effect on the second presentation; and $c_{Fame \times Repetition} = c_{Famous:Rep1>Nonfamous:Rep1} - c_{Famous:Rep2>Nonfamous:Rep2}$, a one-sided test of the interaction, repitition-dependent effect of famousness.

The interaction contrast $c_{Fame \times Repetition}$ is perhaps the most interesting effect, but it detects voxels both where the $c_{Famous:Rep1>Nonfamous:Rep1}$ effect is positive and greater than $c_{Famous:Rep2>Nonfamous:Rep2}$ *and* where decreases in the $c_{Famous:Rep1>Nonfamous:Rep1}$ effect are less negative than decreases in $c_{Famous:Rep2>Nonfamous:Rep2}$. Assume we are only interested in the interaction when the effects of famousness are positive. We can address this by first creating the statistic image for $c_{Famous:Rep1>Nonfamous:Rep1}$ and thresholding at 0 to create a binary mask indicating where $c_{Famous:Rep1>Nonfamous:Rep1}$ is positive. We then create the statistic image for $c_{Fame \times Repetition}$, apply significance thresholding as usual, and finally apply the binary mask. The resulting map will show significant effects for $c_{Fame \times Repetition}$ *masked* for positive effects of famousness. Note that here we are using masking as an image processing manipulation, eliminating voxels that satisfy an arbitrary condition on a supplemental contrast. That is, the statistical threshold is uninformed about the nature of the mask, and, in general, the false positive rate will be only lower after application of such a mask. See the next section for use of regions of interest to change the search region and affect the multiple testing correction.

Whereas an interaction looks for differences in effects, a *conjunction* looks for similarities (Nichols et al., 2005). For example, we may wish to find regions where there is a Fame effect for both the first and second face presentation. A conjunction of the tests specified by contrasts $c_{Famous:Rep1>Nonfamous:Rep1}$ and $c_{Famous:Rep2>Nonfamous:Rep2}$ will provide this inference. Note that this conjunction is *not* the same as the main effect of Fame, $c_{Famous>Nonfamous}$, which could be significant if there was a positive Fame effect in just either the first or second presentation.

Valid conjunction inference is obtained by thresholding each statistic image separately and then taking the voxel-level intersection of above-threshold voxels. There is no assumption of independence between each contrast tested, and the voxel-level significance level of the conjunction is that of each of the combined tests; for example, if a 5% FWE voxel-level threshold is applied to each statistic image, the conjunction inference has level 5% FWE. Alternatively, the voxel-wise minimum can be computed, and this minimum image can be thresholded as if it were a single statistic image. The precise definition of conjunction inference is that it measures the evidence against the *conjunction null hypothesis* that one or more effects are null.

Note there is often low power to detect a conjunction, simply because it is a stringent requirement that each and every test must demonstrate a significant effect. Friston et al. (2005) proposed a weakened form of conjunction inference that also uses the minimum statistic of K effects. Instead of making inference on the conjunction null hypothesis, which has an alternative hypothesis that all K effects are true, they make inference on an intermediate null whose alternative holds that at least $k < K$ of the effects are true. This alternative approach, however, requires an assumption of independence between the tested effects and, as stated, cannot provide an inference that all effects are true.

7.5 Use of region of interest masks

If a study is focused on a particular region of the brain, then it is possible to limit the search for activations to a region of interest, which reduces the stringency of the correction for multiple testing. In Chapter 10 we discuss the issue of ROI analysis in more detail; here we focus on the use of ROIs with voxel-level or cluster-level inference to reduce the volume of brain searched for activations, often known as a 'small volume correction'. The advantage of this strategy is that the ROI definitions do not have to be very precise, as they are only used to define regions of the brain that are of interest or not. As mentioned before, it is crucial that the ROI is defined independently of the statistical analysis of interest.

The only practical concerns to be aware of is that not all multiple testing procedures work equally well for very small ROIs. Cluster-level inference based on RFT, for example, assumes that the search region is large relative to the smoothness of the noise. Clusters that touch the edge of the search can have their significance underestimated, with either RFT or permutation, thus cluster-level inference is not ideal when using ROIs smaller than about 25 RESELs. For example, if FWHM *in voxel units* is $[3, 3, 3]$ voxels^3, a 1,000-voxel ROI has RESEL count $1,000/(3 \times 3 \times 3) = 37.0$, and thus is sufficiently large. Similarly voxel-level inference with FDR correction can work poorly when ROIs are very small. In essence, FDR has to *learn* the distribution of nonnull P-values to distinguish them from the background of null P-values.

7.6 Computing statistical power

One of the most common questions asked of statisticians is "How many subjects do I need in my study in order to detect a hypothesized effect?" To answer this question, we need to compute the *statistical power* of the test. As mentioned at the start of the chapter, power is the probability of correctly rejecting the null hypothesis when it is false (i.e., when there is a true signal). Figure 7.6 illustrates how power is calculated for a simple univariate test. The red distribution is the null distribution of a Z test

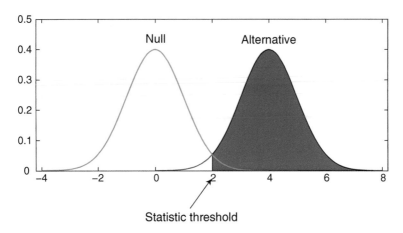

Figure 7.6. Illustration of how power is calculated. The red distribution is the null distribution, which is centered about 0, and the blue distribution is the alternative distribution centered about a value determined by the expected mean and variance of the activation. The statistic threshold indicates the threshold that is used to assess whether or not a statistic value is significant or not. The area under the null distribution to the right of this threshold is the type I error rate, α, and the area under the alternative distribution to the right of this threshold (blue shaded region) is the power.

statistic, and the blue distribution is the alternative distribution. The mean of the alternative distribution is a function of the size of the activation you expect to have in your study, its variance, and the sample size. For a given α level (e.g., $\alpha = 0.05$ for a single test), you find the corresponding null distribution threshold such that the area to the right of this threshold under the null distribution is α (the Type I error rate) and then the area to the right of this threshold under the alternative distribution is the power. If your test has 80% power, it means that you will have, with many possible replicate experiments, an 80% chance of detecting the specified signal.

Power analyses must be carried out *prior* to data collection to plan how many subjects are necessary for a study. The power calculation itself is a function of the number of subjects in the study; the Type I error rate, α; the size of the effect that you wish to be able to detect, δ; and the variance of this effect, σ^2. Power is also impacted by the number of runs of data that will be collected and the length of the runs because those factors affect the variance of the effect (see Mumford & Nichols, 2008, for details). Using this calculation, one can compute the number of subjects necessary to find the desired effect with 80% power, which is the generally accepted threshold for reasonable power. The size of the effect and its variance are often based on pilot data or data from a similar previous study. As discussed in Chapter 6, the variance of the effect takes on a complicated form, including a within-subject and between-subject component, and so it must be carefully estimated to reflect this structure.

In fMRI, we are of course faced with thousands of tests, and thus a comprehensive power analysis would require specifying the effect size of every voxel. Further, the probability calculations would have to account for spatial correlation and the multiple testing problem. In practice this isn't done (though see Hayasaka et al., 2007), and to simplify power analyses we consider only an a priori ROI, and predict the power for the mean percent BOLD change in that ROI based on a simple single-group ordinary least squares (OLS) model. While our aims are rarely so simple, if one doesn't have sufficient power for this setting, any other analysis will surely be underpowered. In this case, the power analysis is simply that of a one-sample t-test. From pilot data, if $\hat{\mu}$ is the ROI mean (over space and subjects) and $\hat{\sigma}$ is the ROI standard deviation (over subjects, of the ROI mean), then the power for a sample size of N and a type I error rate of α would be

$$\text{Power} = P(T_{NCP,N-1} > t_{1-\alpha,N-1}) \qquad (7.2)$$

where $T_{NCP,N-1}$ corresponds to a noncentral T random variable where NCP is the noncentrality parameter and is set to $NCP = \frac{\sqrt{N}\hat{\mu}}{\hat{\sigma}}$ and $t_{1-\alpha,N-1}$ is the $1-\alpha$ quantile of a central t distribution with $N-1$ degrees of freedom. For other group models such as a two-sample t-test or ANOVA, models estimated using OLS examples can be found in Cohen (1988), and estimation techniques for full mixed effects models can be found in Mumford & Nichols (2008). A tool for computing power estimates based on previous studies is also available at http://www.fmripower.org.

As an example, say you are planning a new study using a stop signal task and want to ensure you have sufficient subjects to distinguish between successfully stopping versus not successfully stopping in the putamen. You have a previous study with data on 16 subjects for this very sort of experiment and contrast; by using this data we make the assumption that our future study will use a similar scanner and acquisition parameters, preprocessing options, number of trials per run, and runs per subject. Using an anatomical atlas to create a mask for the putamen, we measure the mean BOLD signal change in for each subject (see Section 10.4.3.3 for instructions on converting to percent signal change units). We find that the mean over subjects is 0.8% BOLD signal change units, and the standard deviation across subjects is 2% BOLD. Based on these two numbers and α-level 0.05 using a range of sample sizes with Equation 7.2, the power curve in Figure 7.7 is generated. This curve crosses the 80% mark between 40 and 41 subjects and so a sample of at least 41 subjects will yield at least 80% power, if the given effect is 0.8% and standard deviation is 2%. Note, if you are working on a grant application the power calculations will often not be what you had hoped and you will need to refigure your budget. Because of this, carrying out your power analyses well in advance of your grant deadline is highly recommended.

Several limitations of power analyses are worth considering. First and foremost, appreciate that power computations are quite speculative enterprises. The whole

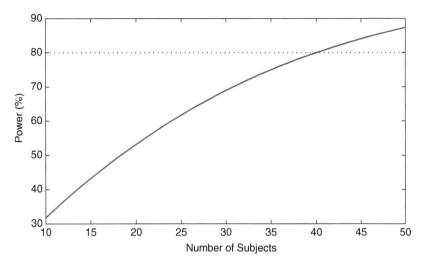

Figure 7.7.   Power curve. The curve was generated using an estimated mean effect of 0.8% signal change units with standard deviation of 2% signal change units and a type I error rate of 0.05 using Equation 7.2. Since the graph crosses 80% between 40 and 41 subjects, a sample size of 41 will yield at least 80% power.

point of planning an experiment is to study an effect, yet a power analysis assumes you know the true effect magnitude and standard deviation. Thus, it is a good idea to consider a range of "what if" scenarios: What if the true effect is 10% smaller? 20% smaller? What if standard deviation is off, by 10%? and so on. If it appears you still have good power over a range of alternative scenarios, you should be in good shape.

Second, never compute the power of a study post hoc. That is, it is pointless to assess the power of a study that has already been performed: If the effect is there and you detect it, you have 100% power; if it is there and you missed it, you have 0% power. Another way to see this is to consider a series of failed experiments, where the null hypothesis is always true. If $\alpha = 0.05$ is used, we will reject the null hypothesis and declare a significant result on 5% of these tests. Further, say the observed test statistic t is just equal to the statistic threshold, and we use t to compute an effect size and power (t could be higher, but let's be pessimistic). In this case, you will compute the power to be 50% (as it can be inferred from Figure 7.6, if you shift the mean of the alternative distribution left to equal the statistic threshold). Thus, a series of failed experiments will tell you that you have at least 50% power whenever they detect something, when in fact you have 0% power.

Finally, best practice dictates that you base your power analysis on studies that are as similar to your planned study as possible. From those studies, calculate the typical mean and standard deviation of the relevant effect and use independently determined ROIs to avoid circular estimates of effect size (see Box 10.4.2). For more details on the limitations of power analysis, see Hoenig & Heisey (2001).

Modeling brain connectivity

8.1 Introduction

One of the oldest debates in the history of neuroscience centers on the localization of function in the brain; that is, whether specific mental functions are localized to specific brain regions or instead rely more diffusely upon the entire brain (Finger, 1994). The concept of localization first arose from work by Franz Gall and the phrenologists, who attempted to localize mental functions to specific brain regions based on the shape of the skull. Although Gall was an outstanding neuroscientist (Zola-Morgan, 1995), he was wrong in his assumption about how the skull relates to the brain, and phrenology was in the end taken over by charlatans. In the early twentieth century, researchers such as Karl Lashley argued against localization of function, on the basis of research showing that cortical lesions in rats had relatively global effects on behavior. However, across the twentieth century the pendulum shifted toward a localizationist view, such that most neuroscientists now agree that there is at least some degree of localization of mental function. At the same time, the function of each of these regions must be integrated in order to acheive coherent mental function and behavior. These concepts have been referred to as *functional specialization* and *functional integration*, respectively (Friston, 1994).

Today, nearly all neuroimaging studies are centered on functional localization. However, there is increasing recognition that neuroimaging research must take functional integration seriously to fully explain brain function (Friston, 2005; McIntosh, 2000). This chapter outlines methods for analyzing brain connectivity with fMRI data, which provide a means to understand how spatially distant brain regions interact and work together to create mental function. Whereas the methods in the foregoing chapters reflect a general consensus about how fMRI data should be analyzed, there is much less agreement about how brain connectivity should be analyzed, and these methods are undergoing continual development and refinement. We attempt to provide a broad overview of the extant methods, focusing on those for which there are available implementations for fMRI data.

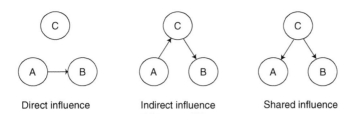

Figure 8.1.   A depiction of the various ways in which correlated activity between two regions A and B can arise, either through direct influence (left panel), indirect influence via another region (center panel), or shared influence of a common input region (right panel).

8.2 Functional connectivity

Functional connectivity refers to correlations in activity between spatially remote brain regions, which can arise for a number of reasons (see Figure 8.1). First, it could reflect the direct influence of one region on another, which is known as *effective connectivity* (see Section 8.3). For example, if one region sends efferent connections to another, then signals along those connections could result in correlated activity in the two regions. Second, it could reflect the influence of another region that is mediated by a third region. Third, it could reflect a common input to both regions. For example, if two different regions both receive inputs from the visual cortex, then presentation of visual stimuli will cause activity that is correlated between those regions, even if they do not directly influence one another. This has been referred to as the problem of stimulus-driven transients. The critical point is that only in the first case does functional connectivity reflect a direct causal influence between regions. For this reason, results from functional connectivity analyses must be interpreted with great care.

8.2.1 Seed voxel correlation: Between-subjects

Perhaps the simplest approach that has sometimes been used to examine connectivity is to measure the correlation in activation (e.g., contrast values or parameter estimates) across subjects. In this approach, some estimate of activation (e.g., beta weights for a particular condition) are extracted for a particular region, and then those values are entered into a whole-brain regression analysis across subjects. The intuition behind this approach is that if two regions are functionally connected, then they should show similarly varying levels of activity across subjects. However, this approach is severely limited by the fact that between-subject correlations across regions need not reflect any kind of functional connectivity. As an example, imagine a case where two different regions receive input from visual cortex, but their activity is independent and uncorrelated within each subject. However, subjects differ in their overall amount of activation (e.g., due to whether they drank coffee prior to the scan). In this case, there will be a significant correlation between these regions across subjects, even when there is no correlation within subjects. Such spurious correlations can occur if some subjects show greater BOLD response than others due to noise (e.g., subjects who move more may show smaller activation signals) or physiological factors (e.g., recent ingestion of caffiene or tobacco). These possibilities suggest that positive correlation between regional activation across subjects must be interpreted with caution. It may be the case that negative correlations are more interpretable because they unlikely reflect the kind of global factors that were outlined earlier. Between-subjects correlation may provide interesting data to complement other forms of connectivity analysis (cf. McIntosh, 1999), but it is likely to be insufficient to establish connectivity on its own.

8.2.2 Seed voxel correlation: Within-subjects

Another simple way to estimate functional connectivity is to compute the correlation between the timecourses of different regions. This is most often done by first extracting the timecourse from a *seed voxel* or *seed region*, which is determined based on some a priori hypothesis, and then computing its correlation with all of the voxels across the brain. When extracting signal from a region, one can either take the mean of the voxels at each point in the timecourse or extract the first eigenvariate of the region (as in done in SPM). The first eigenvariate reflects the component of variance that accounts for the most variance in the signal and that is orthogonal to all other components (see Section 8.2.5.1 for more on this idea). The rationale for using this method rather than the mean is that if there are mulitple signal sources within the region, the first eigenvariate will reflect the strongest single source whereas the mean will reflect a combination of multiple sources. In practice there appears to be very little difference between these methods.

Box 8.2.2. An example dataset for connectivity analysis

For all of the approaches described in this chapter, we will use the same dataset (which is availale for download on the book Web site, along with instructions to complete the example analyses).

The data in this example are from a subject (randomly selected from a larger group) performing rhyming judgments on either words or pseudowords across separate blocks (Xue & Poldrack, unpublished data). On each trial, the subject judged whether a pair of visually presented stimuli rhymed or not by pressing one of two response keys. In each 20-second block, eight pairs of words were presented for 2.5 seconds each. Blocks were separated by 20-second periods of visual fixation. Four blocks of words were followed by four blocks of pseudowords.

The data were acquired on a Siemens Allegra 3T MRI scanner, using the following scanning parameters: $TR = 2000$ ms, $TE = 30$ ms, field of view $= 200$ mm, matrix size $= 64 \times 64$, 33 slices, slice thickness $= 4$ mm (0 skip), 160 timepoints.

8.2.2.1 Avoiding activation-induced correlations

If correlations are computed in a whole-brain manner across an entire timecourse, then most regions that are activated by the task will be correlated due to this shared activation effect, even if there is no functional connectivity between them. There are two ways to address this issue.

The first approach, which is suitable for blocked design fMRI studies only, is to extract the timepoints from within blocks for each condition and then concatenate those timepoints, so that one obtains a timecourse that reflects each single condition. To account for the delay in fMRI response, it is necessary to remove the first few timepoints (about 6 seconds worth of data) from each block. This method has been used successfully to examine differences in connectivity across conditions (e.g., Bokde et al., 2001).

The second approach, which is suitable for any fMRI design, involves first fitting a model that includes the task as well as any other parameters that might account for systematic variance in the data (e.g., motion parameters), as one would generally do in a first-level analysis. Because this model is meant to remove variance that we are not interested in for the connectivity analysis, it is referred to as a *nuisance model* in this context. After this model is estimated, the residuals from the model can be obtained, and these residuals are then analyzed for their correlation with the seed region, by entering the residuals from the seed region as a regressor in the model. Because any misspecification of the model can result in structured variance that could cause activation effects in the correlation analysis, it is important that the nuisance model includes any possible source of variance as well as including temporal derivatives to account for timing misspecification.

8.2.3 Beta-series correlation

Another way to address the problem of activation-induced correlations is to estimate the size of the evoked response on each trial separately at each voxel and then to examine the correlation of these responses, rather than the correlation in the entire timecourse. Figure 8.2 shows an example of the technique known as *beta-series correlation* (Rissman et al., 2004), in which the response to each event is estimated (or *deconvolved*) by fitting a model that includes a separate regressor for each trial. The correlation in the parameter estimates on these regressors (the "beta series") between regions provides a means of examining the degree to which they show similar trial-by-trial fluctuations, as would be expected if they are functionally connected.

The beta-series model can be usefully applied to event-related fMRI studies where the spacing between trials is relatively long (greater than 8–10 seconds). With faster designs, the overlap in hemodynamic responses between subsequent trials can cause correlations within the design matrix that can result in highly variable parameter estimates. While it is possible in theory to use regularized methods such as ridge

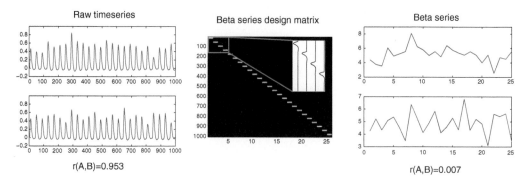

Figure 8.2.   Beta-series correlation estimates a response for each trial using a separate regressor, as shown in the design matrix in the middle of the figure. The original timeseries for the two regions plotted in the figure are highly correlated ($r = 0.953$), due to activation-related transients in the signal. When the beta series is estimated using the general linear model with the design matrix shown in the middle, the resulting estimates show that the trial-by-trial response of these two regions is actually uncorrelated ($r = 0.007$). Thus, beta-series correlation can identify functional connectivity without being sensitive to activation-induced effects.

regression to estimate such models (Rizk-Jackson et al., 2008), there is likely to be a substantial loss in power. Thus, this method is most appropriate for relatively slow event-related designs.

8.2.4 Psychophysiological interaction

The foregoing approaches allow estimation of correlations that extend across an entire imaging run (i.e., that do not change with the task). However, the question of interest is often how functional connectivity is modulated by a task. The first method described earlier, involving dicing of the timecourse into task-specific sections, allows this question to be asked, but it requires comparison of correlations across runs which can be problematic.

A more elegant way to ask the question of how connectivity with a seed region is modulated by some other factor (such as a task) is the *psychophysiological interaction* (PPI) approach (Friston et al., 1997). In PPI, the standard GLM modeling the task at the first level is used along with an additional regressor that models the interaction between the task and the timecourse in a seed voxel. For example, for a model with a single task regressor (X), the standard GLM would be

$$Y = \beta_0 + \beta_1 X + \epsilon$$

For the PPI analysis, the model would also include regressors that model the signal from the seed region (R) and the interaction between the seed region and the task:

$$Y = \beta_0 + \beta_1 X + \beta_2 R + \beta_3 R * X + \epsilon$$

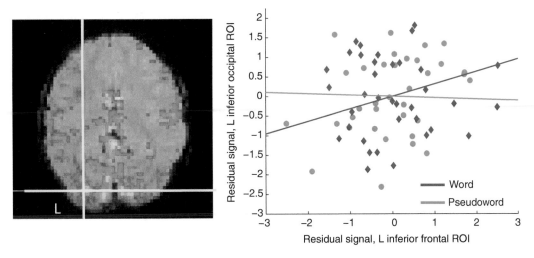

Figure 8.3.   Comparison of PPI and seed voxel correlation results. The left panel shows the results from a PPI analysis on the example dataset; regions showing in color had a significant PPI reflecting greater connectivity with a seed region in the left prefrontal cortex during processing of words versus pseudowords. The right panel shows the results of separate seed voxel correlation analyses using the nuisance model approach. Timepoints from the word blocks are shown in blue and those from the pseudoword blocks are shown in red, with regression lines for each in the same color. The X axis is signal from the left prefrontal seed voxel, and the Y axis is signal from the left inferior occipital region (denoted by yellow crosshairs in the left image). There was a small but significant linear relation between activity in these regions during the word blocks but no such relation in the pseudoword blocks.

A positive effect for the interaction regressor β_3 reflects the modulation of the slope of the linear relation with the seed voxel depending upon the variable used to create the interaction. For example, in Figure 8.3, we see that the slope between the left inferior frontal cortex and the lateral inferior temporal cortex is greater when the subject performs a rhyming task with words compared to the same task with pseudowords.

8.2.4.1 Creating the PPI regressor

In the approach described previously, the PPI regressor was created by multiplying the BOLD timecourse of the region of interest with the task regressor. However, our goal is to create a regressor that reflects neuronal activity at each timepoint, which is going to be smeared out in the raw fMRI data. This is of particular concern for event-related fMRI studies, where trials from different conditions may overlap in time, resulting in contributions from different conditions at each timepoint in the fMRI signal. A solution to this problem was proposed by Gitelman et al. (2003), which involves estimation of the underlying neuronal signal from the observed fMRI signal using *deconvolution*. In essence, deconvolution determines the most likely neuronal signal that could have given rise to the observed fMRI signal, taking into account the nature of the hemodynamic response (Glover, 1999).

The approach of Gitelman et al. (2003) uses a large set of basis functions to model the neuronal signal, so many that the design matrix has as many regressors as timepoints. Specifically, if y was the BOLD seed voxel timeseries that we were interested in obtaining the neuronal signal for and if H is the HRF matrix, the model used would be $y = HB\beta + \epsilon$, where **B** is a *square* design matrix comprised of as many basis functions as timepoints. The reason so many regressors are used is to have as much flexibility as possible to capture the shape of the neuronal response. Once $\hat{\beta}$ is obtained, the neuronal signal estimate is simply $B\hat{\beta}$. Although using such a large set of basis functions will allow for the most flexible fit of the neuronal signal, the estimates for a linear model with a square design matrix are very unstable. Typically, this problem can be solved by simply removing unnecessary regressors from the design. For example, we'd expect the neuronal response to be relatively smooth, so removing high-frequency basis functions could be considered, but this would sacrifice the quality of the fit. A solution is to use a regularized model estimation technique, which imposes prior assumptions on the shape of the response. In this case, for example, higher-frequency basis functions would be down-weighted through priors in a Bayesian estimation procedure. This is more appealing than simply removing higher-frequency trends, since higher-frequency trends aren't completely removed. Once the signal is deconvolved, then the PPI regressor is created by multiplying the unconvolved task regressor by the deconvolved signal regressor $(B\hat{\beta})$, and then this is reconvolved in order to place it back into the hemodynamic domain.

8.2.4.2 Potential problems with PPI

One problem that can occur with PPI, especially in event-related designs, is that the PPI regressor may be highly correlated with the task regressor. If the task regressor is not included, then any activation observed for the PPI cannot be uniquely attributed to the interaction, as it could also reflect the overall effect of the task. For this reason, the task regressor and seed regressor should always be included in the statistical model for a PPI analysis alongside the PPI regressor. However, if both task and PPI regressors are included in the model, then this can result in a lack of efficiency due to the variance inflation that occurs with correlated regressors. Thus, the correlation between PPI and task regressors should always be examined, and if it is too high, then the results should be treated with caution.

Another problem with PPI is that it assumes that the fit of the hemodynamic model is exact. If there is any misspecification of the model, then this could drive correlations that reflect activation-induced effects rather than reflecting functional connectivity.

8.2.5 Multivariate decomposition

There are a number of ways to decompose a matrix into separate components, which can be used to identify coherently active networks from fMRI data. In the language of matrix algebra, these are known as *matrix factorization* methods. Each

Principal components analysis   Independent components analysis

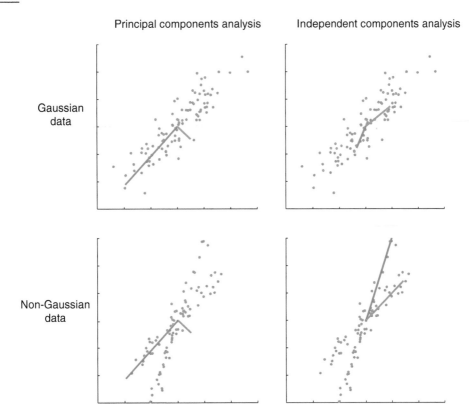

Figure 8.4. PCA and ICA find different types of structure in the data. In the top panel, the data are sampled from a Gaussian distribution. The two components detected by each technique are shown as red and green lines. With Gaussian data, PCA finds the direction with the most variance as the first component, and the orthogonal direction as the second component (top left). ICA finds a different set of components with this dataset, which likely reflects fitting to the noise since there is no signal remaining once the data have been whitened (top right). In the lower panel, the data are a mixture of two different signals. PCA cannot find these sources of variance since they are not orthogonal (bottom left), whereas ICA is able to accurately detect the two signals in the data (bottom right).

of these methods assumes that the data are composed of some number of underlying components that are mixed together to form the observed data. The main differences between methods center on how the underlying components are related to one another and how they are estimated from the data.

8.2.5.1 Principal components analysis

One of best-known methods for matrix decomposition is principal components analysis (PCA). PCA is a method for reexpressing a dataset in terms of a set of components that are uncorrelated, or *orthogonal* to one another. As shown in Figure 8.4, the first principal component is equivalent to the direction through the data that has the greatest amount of variance; the second principal component is the direction that accounts for the next greatest amount of variance and is uncorrelated with the first principal component, and so on. The number of components is the minimum of the number of dimensions or observations; in fMRI data, there are generally many more dimensions (voxels) than there are observations (timepoints or subjects). PCA can also be used as a *data reduction* technique; for example, instead of analyzing the data from each of the thousands of voxels in the brain, one might analyze the data from just the first few principal components, which account for the majority of the variance in the data. This is discussed further in Section 9.4 regarding machine learning analyses.

To perform PCA on fMRI data, the data must be reformatted into a two-dimensional matrix, with voxels as columns and timepoints/subjects as rows. PCA will provide a set of components that have a value for each timepoint, which reflects the combinations of voxels that account for the most variance. Each of these components also has a loading for each voxel, which denotes how much that voxel contributes to each component. Figure 8.5 shows an example of some PCA components for the example dataset.

PCA was used as a method for functional connectivity analysis in some early studies (Friston et al., 1993). It has the benefit of being simple and easily implemented. However, it has the substantial drawback of being sensitive only to signals that follow a Gaussian distribution. Although some signals in fMRI data clearly do follow such a distribution (as shown in Figure 8.5), there are many signals of interest that will be mixed together by PCA because they do not follow a Gaussian distribution. In this case, independent components analysis is a more appropriate technique, and in practice ICA has largely supplanted PCA as a method for characterizing functional connectivity.

8.2.5.2 Independent components analysis

Independent components analysis was developed to solve the problem of detecting unknown signals in a dataset, sometimes called the *blind source separation* problem. This problem is often described using the example of a cocktail party (Hyvärinen & Oja, 2000). Imagine a party with microphones placed throughout the room and a large number of people talking. A blind source separation problem would be to separate out the speech stream of each person speaking using only the recordings from these microphones. The idea is that the recording from each microphone reflects a mixture of all of the different speakers (weighted by their distance from the microphone, their head direction, etc.), and our goal is to *unmix* the sources from the recordings; we assume that the speakers and microphones do not move during the recording, so that the mixing process is stationary during the recording.

Formally, the ICA model is defined as

$$x = As$$

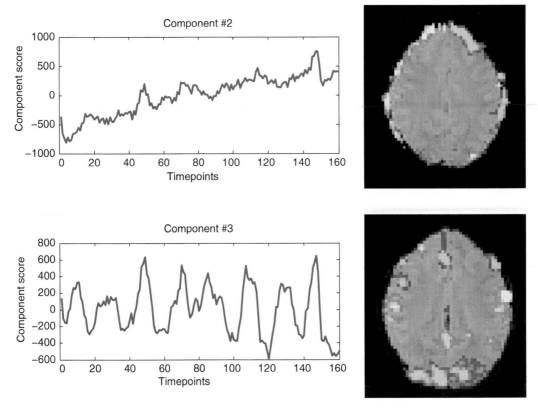

Figure 8.5. PCA applied to the example dataset. The right panels show the voxels that load strongly on two particular PCA components (red: positive loading, blue: negative loading), and the left panels show the timecourse of each component. Component #2 has the hallmarks of slow sideways motion, as highlighted by positive loading on one side and negative loading on the other side of the brain along with a slowly drifting timecourse. Component #3 appears to be task-related in its timecourse and shows positive loading in the frontal lobes bilaterally.

where x is the signal that we are trying to decompose, s is a set of unkonwn sources (or *components*), and A is the unknown *mixing matrix* that combines the components to obtain the observed signal.

Because both A and s are both unknown, we have to make some assumptions if we are to be able to find a unique solution to the problem, and in general we will make assumptions about the relation between the different components in s. If we assume that they are orthogonal and Gaussian, then we can solve the problem using PCA. However, if the signals from the different sources are not orthogonal and Gaussian (as is likely in cases like the cocktail party example) then PCA will not be able to find them.

ICA relies upon the assumption that the components in s are *statistically independent*. Statistical independence of two signals *A* and *B* obtains when the joint

Box 8.2.5. Resting state fMRI

The initial development of fMRI was driven by researchers interested in under-standing the brain's evoked responses to external events or mental stimuli. Thus, nearly all research focused on the measurement of responses evoked by con-trolled tasks inspired by cognitive psychology. However, two early findings drove researchers to move away from this sole focus on task-evoked activity. First, it became clear that there is a set of brain regions whose activity is high at rest and almost invariably goes down whenever one performs a demanding cognitive task (Shulman et al., 1997). In fact, most experienced fMRI researchers would agree that this decrease of activity in regions including the ventromedial prefrontal cor-tex, precuneus, and temporoparietal cortex is the most replicable finding in all neuroimaging research! Marcus Raichle and his colleagues (Raichle et al., 2001) proposed that this activity reflects what they called the brain's "default mode," which they proposed to reflect the true metabolic baseline of brain activity.

Second, Biswal et al. (1995) published a study in which subjects simply rested in the scanner, and the data were then examined using a seed correlation analysis with a seed in the left motor cortex. This analysis found that other regions in the motor system (including the thalamus and contralateral motor cortex) showed correlations with the seed, suggesting that correlations in resting state activity can provide insight into the function of neural systems even if they are not actively engaged. Subsequent work has shown that resting-state fMRI data contains a great deal of interesting structure, to the degree that one can detect many of the same networks that are engaged during different kinds of cognitive tasks in addition to default-mode regions (Smith et al., 2009). This work shows that it is essential to distinguish resting-state and default-mode concepts, since the default mode is only one of the networks that appears in resting state FMRI data.

Since about 2000, there has been an explosion in the use of resting-state fMRI to characterize brain function. Many of these studies have used ICA (Section 8.2.5.2) because of its ability to robustly detect networks of coherent activity during rest. Others have used the network analysis approaches described in Section 8.4, or seed correlation analyses designed to identify the correlates of specific regions at rest.

probability is equal to the product of the individual probabilities: $P(A, B) = P(A)P(B)$. When A and B are independent, then knowing the value of one does not provide any information about the value of the other. In cases where the signal components are generated by independent processes (such as independent speakers at a cocktail party, or independent neural processes in fMRI), ICA may be more able than PCA to correctly identify the component sources because they will likely be non-Gaussian.

Independence is related to but different from orthogonality (or uncorrelatedness); it is possible that two variables can be statistically dependent even if they are orthogonal, which occurs when the data do not conform to a Gaussian distribution. In fact, the independent components in ICA are estimated by searching for non-Gaussian signals in the data. The details of ICA estimation are beyond the scope of this book, but the interested reader should consult Hyvärinen & Oja (2000) for an overview. Since ICA searches for non-Gaussian signals, most ICA algorithms first *whiten* the data using PCA in order to remove any Gaussian signals in the data. Some software packages (e.g., FSL's MELODIC) will output both the PCA and ICA results, and it may be useful to examine both in order to retain sensitivity to the widest range of signals in the data.

The standard ICA model is "noise-free," since it does not include an error term to represent the noise in the data. A probabilistic ICA model has been developed (Beckmann & Smith, 2004) that includes a noise term:

$$\mathbf{x} = \mathbf{As} + \mathbf{e}$$

where $\mathbf{e} \sim N(0, \sigma)$. This model has the advantage of allowing statistical inference on the estimated sources, by providing measures of error for the estimated components and parameters. The probabilistic ICA model is implemented in the MELODIC software in FSL .

To apply ICA to fMRI data, the data must first be rearranged into a two-dimensional matrix. When applying ICA to fMRI timecourse data, it is necessary to choose whether the algorithm should search for components that are either spatially independent or temporally independent (which is determined by which way the input matrix is oriented). Most methods have assumed spatially independent components; when applied in this way, ICA returns a set of spatial components along with a mixing matrix that denotes the contribution of each spatial pattern to the observed signal at each timepoint (as shown in Figure 8.6). The assumption of spatial independence can be justified based on the intuition that there is a large number of potentially independent networks in the brain, which might have similar timecourses during performance of a task. It provides the ability to detect spatially distinct effects (such as task activation versus task-correlated head motion) that may have correlated timecourses.

There are a number of qualifications that must be kept in mind when using ICA. First, ICA solutions are not unique, and thus require additional constraints to determine an optimal solution. Some of these methods, such as the probabilistic ICA model in FSL, are stochastic, such that different solutions may occur when the same dataset is run multiple times through the ICA procedure. Second, because it is sensitive to non-Gaussian structure, ICA can be very sensitive to outliers in the data. This is generally seen as a positive, since it makes ICA useful for identifying

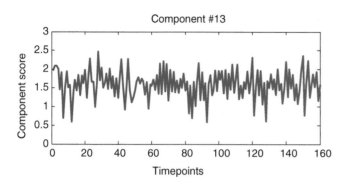

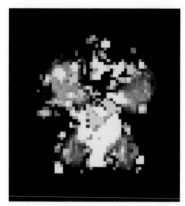

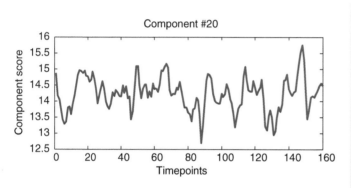

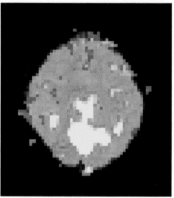

Figure 8.6.   ICA applied to the example dataset. The top panels show data from a component that appears to represent high-frequency oscillations, most likely due to cardiac pulsation. This component loaded most heavily in the most inferior slices covering the brain stem, as shown in the slice image. The bottom panels show a component that has a potentially task-relevant waveform and show heaviest loading in the medial parietal and intraparietal regions. ICA was performed using using the FastICA toolbox for MATLAB.

potential artifacts, but in the context of finding connected networks it is important to ensure that the results are not driven by outliers.

8.2.5.3 Performing ICA/PCA on group data

As with univariate analyses, we often perform connectivity analyses with the intent of finding patterns that are consistent across individuals rather than idiosyncratic to any particular person. However, combining the results from ICA or PCA analyses across subjects is complicated by the fact that there is no simple way to match components across individuals, since they do not have any natural ordering. For example, one subject may have a component that reflects task-driven activation as #13, whereas for another subject this component may be #2.

There are a number of ways in which group ICA/PCA analysis has been performed (Calhoun et al., 2009). Perhaps the simplest is to average the data across subjects and then perform ICA on the mean dataset. This has the advantage of being simple, but it will only provide power to find components that are highly consistent across individuals in both time and space; any idiosyncratic effects are likely to be averaged away. This approach also does not work to detect resting state signals (Box 8.2.5), since they will largely be temporally uncorrelated across individuals. Another approach is to perform ICA on each individual, and then use some form of clustering or correlation analysis to match components between individuals. While intuitively appealing, the noisiness of the estimated components can make it difficult to accurately match components across individuals. A slightly more sophisticated approach is to concatenate the data matrices for each individual (after spatial normalization to align voxels across individuals). Concatenating across time will result in detection of shared spatial components, whereas concatenation across voxels will result in detection of shared timecourses across individuals. Most studies have used concatenation across time, and a comparison of these different methods using simulated data suggested that concatenating across time is more reliable than averaging over subjects or concatenating across voxels (Schmithorst & Holland, 2004).

There are several ways to estimate the timecourses of the spatially independent components (i.e., the mixing matrix) when data are concatenated across time. In the GIFT software (Calhoun et al., 2009), a separate mixing matrix is estimated for each individual. In the Tensor–PICA approach implemented in FSL (Beckmann & Smith, 2005), a common group mixing matrix is estimated, and a scaling factor is estimated for each subject. Because it assumes a common timecourse, the Tensor–PICA approach is less suitable for cases where the timecourses may differ across individuals, such as in resting-state fluctuations. Other approaches are also available that fall in between these methods (Guo & Pagnoni, 2008).

8.2.6 Partial least squares

The foregoing methods for matrix decomposition focused on decomposing the fMRI data, without regard to any other knowledge that one might have, such as knowledge about a task or some measurement such as behavioral performance. Partial least squares (PLS) is a method that simultaneously decomposes the fMRI data and a design matrix in a way that maximizes the covariance between them. Thus, whereas PCA and ICA find components that explain the most variance in the data alone, PLS finds components that best explain the relation between the data and the design matrix (Abdi, 2003). PLS was first applied to PET data (McIntosh et al., 1996) and later to fMRI data. When applied to neuroimaging data, the design matrix can either reflect a task manipulation (i.e., the same design matrix used in the standard

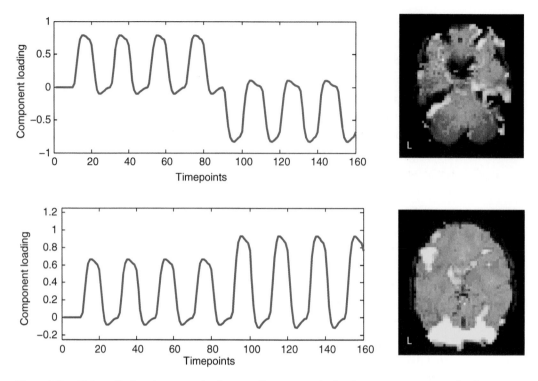

Figure 8.7.   PLS applied to the example dataset. The top row is the first PLS component; its timecourse reflects a larger response to the first four blocks (the word condition) compared to the second four blocks (the pseudoword condition). The spatial pattern of this component, which closely follows the brain outline in the lower slice shown in the figure, suggests that it likely reflects a task-related motion artifact that subsided over the run. The second row is the second component, which loads roughly equally for both tasks and shows engagement of regions known to be involved in reading. (Thanks to Herve Abdi for the MATLAB code used to create this figure.)

GLM analysis) or possibly behavioral performance associated with each observation (McIntosh & Lobaugh, 2004). For example, in Figure 8.7, PLS was performed on the example dataset using the design matrix containing two conditions (as described in Box 8.2.2).

8.3 Effective connectivity

The functional connectivity methods described in the previous section provide evidence regarding how activity covaries across brain regions, and thus can elucidate to some degree the interactions that occur between regions. However, in the end we would often like to make stronger claims; in particular, we would like to know whether activity in one region has a causal influence on activity in another region.

Effective connectivity models attempt to bridge this explanatory gap by providing the ability to test causal models regarding the interactions between regions.

The astute reader may at this point say: "But wait, one of the basic lessons in my first statistics class is that correlation does not equal causation." It is indeed true that correlation between two variables does not necessarily imply a direct causal relation between those variables. However, the presence of a correlation implies that there is a causal relation somewhere (either between the two variables, or via some unmeasured third variable, as seen in Figure 8.1), and correlations most certainly can provide evidence regarding potential causal relations, especially when there are more than two variables. There is now a well-developed theory of causality that has been developed within the machine learning field (Spirtes et al., 2000; Pearl, 2000), which provides mathematical proof that it is possible to test causal hypotheses using only observational data (such as observed correlations). The methods described below take advantage of correlations to extract information and test hypotheses about causal relations between brain regions.

Models of causal processes such as effective connectivity are often expressed in terms of directed graphs, like those shown in Figure 8.1; these are also referred to as *path diagrams* in the context of path analysis and SEM. The *nodes* (circles) in the graph refer to brain areas, and the *edges* (lines with arrows) refer to causal relations. In general, the methods used for effective connectivity analysis are limited to relatively small numbers of variables; for fMRI, these variables are usually the averaged signal within a set of regions of interest.

8.3.1 Challenges to causal inference with fMRI data

There are a number of aspects of fMRI data that render the inference of causal relations very challenging (Ramsey et al., 2010). Here we outline several of the major problems.

Size of the model space.   Given some set of brain regions, the goal of effective connectivity analysis is to understand how those regions influence one another. One obvious approach to answering this question is to test all possible graphs to determine which one best fits the data. However, the number of possible directed graphs increases super-exponentially as a function of the number of regions in the graph; for example, for a graph with six nodes, there are more than one billion possible directed graphs! Even with fast computers, this combinatorial explosion renders exhaustive search of the space impossible for more than about six regions. Another approach that has been taken to this problem is to specify a small set of models based on other knowledge (e.g., knowledge about connectivity from animal models). Although it is possible to reliably compare the fit of a small set of models, the results will only be valid if the most accurate model is contained in the set of tested models, which seems unlikely for large search spaces. Thus, the ability to search for the best possible model amongst the enormous number of alternatives is crucial. Fortunately, there are methods available that make this problem tractable under particular assumptions, which we discuss in Section 8.3.3.

Indirect measurements.   Analyses of effective connectivity are applied to fMRI data, but the causal relations that we wish to discover regard the underlying neuronal signals. Thus, the variables amongst which we wish to model causality are *latent*, or unobserved, and we have to estimate their causal relations from observed signals that include both noise and systematic distortions of the signal (such as hemodynamic delays). Unfortunately, this can result in serious problems for estimating the underlying causal relations. First, it can be shown that measurement noise in the observed measurements (which is substantial for fMRI data) results in the identification of spurious causal relations that do not exist between the latent variables (Ramsey et al., 2010). Second, any differences in the hemodynamic response (e.g., its latency) across regions can also result in the identification of spurious causal relations if one relies upon temporal information to infer causal relations. A number of methods have been proposed to address these problems, which are outlined in the following sections.

Combining data across individuals.   The analysis of effective connectivity is generally performed on timeseries data, which contain relevant information about relations between activation across regions. However, as with activation analyses, we are generally interested in making inferences about the connectivity patterns that exist in the larger population, as opposed to the specific set of individuals sampled. Further, it is likely that the true pattern of connectivity varies across individuals as a function of age, experience, genetics, and other factors; even if they share the same causal structure, the parameters describing connectivity are likely to vary. It is thus important to employ methods that can adequately characterize effective connectivity at the population level. The simplest possible approach would be to simply combine the data across individuals and assess the model on this composite dataset. However, as discussed by Ramsey et al. (2010), pooling data across individuals can lead to an observed pattern of independence and conditional independence relations that are not reflective of any particular individual in the group. Thus, it is necessary to employ some form of "random effects" analysis to ensure that connectivity is properly estimated across the group.

8.3.2 Path analysis and structural equation modeling

The first method proposed for analysis of effective connectivity in neuroimaging was path analysis, which is a form of *structural equation modeling (SEM)*. Introductions to this method can be found in Shipley (2000) and Bentler & Stein (1992), and a formal treatment can be found in Bollen (1989). Because path analysis is a special case of SEM in which there are no unobserved (or *latent*) variables, our discussion will be framed in terms of the more general SEM.

8.3.2.1 Specifying a structural model

SEM is a method by which one can test hypotheses about causal influence between variables. It requires that one start with a model that specifies the hypothesized causal relations, which are specified in terms of a set of linear equations (though it is also possible to create nonlinear structural equation models). For example, take the three variables in Figure 8.1. The relations between these variables can be specified in terms of the following linear equations:

$$A = \beta_{1,1} A + \beta_{1,2} B + \beta_{1,3} C$$
$$B = \beta_{2,1} A + \beta_{2,2} B + \beta_{2,3} C$$
$$C = \beta_{3,1} A + \beta_{3,2} B + \beta_{3,3} C$$

or in matrix notation:

$$
\begin{bmatrix} A \\ B \\ C \end{bmatrix} = \begin{bmatrix} \beta_{1,1} & \beta_{1,2} & \beta_{1,3} \\ \beta_{2,1} & \beta_{2,2} & \beta_{2,3} \\ \beta_{3,1} & \beta_{3,2} & \beta_{3,3} \end{bmatrix} \begin{bmatrix} A \\ B \\ C \end{bmatrix}
$$

We will refer to the matrix of βs as the *connectivity matrix* since it expresses the connectivity between the different variables. The connectivity matrix maps directly to a representation as a directed graph, as shown in Figure 8.8.

In addition to modeling connectivity between regions, an SEM can also include extraneous variables (e.g., which model the task inputs) as well as error terms for the observed variables, as well as *latent* variables, which are hypothesized but unobserved variables that are related in some way to the observed variables (see Section 8.3.2.3 below for more on the role of latent variables in SEM with fMRI).

8.3.2.2 Estimating and testing an SEM

In most of the methods described so far in this book, parameters of statistical models have been estimated by minimizing the difference between the actual data and model predictions. However, SEM uses a different approach. Instead of comparing the actual and predicted data, the parameters in an SEM are estimated by minimizing the difference between the actual and predicted covariance between the variables. The estimated parameters are known as *path coefficients* and represent how much of a change in one variable would occur due to a change in the other variable, holding all other variables constant.

Once the model is estimated, we must use a statistical test to determine how well it fits the observed data. First, it is possible to test the overall fit of the model by examining how well it explains the observed covariances, using a chi-squared test to determine whether the predicted covariance structure is significantly different from the actual structure. Note that this turns the standard hypothesis-testing logic

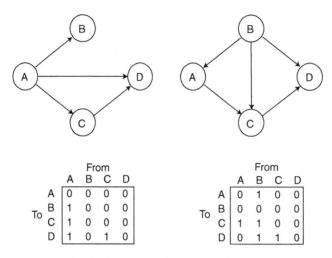

Figure 8.8. Examples of path diagrams and their associated connectivity matrices. In this example, all paths have a strength of either 1 (present) or zero (absent).

on its head: Whereas the null hypothesis is usually the hypothesis that we want to overturn, in this case the null hypothesis is that the model is correct. It is thus critical to understand that a nonsignificant chi-squared test does not imply that the model is true or best, just that we can't reject the hypothesis that it is correct. There could well be many other models that would fit equally well or better. For this reason, the absolute fit of a model is generally not of primary interest.

More often, we wish to test hypotheses about which of a set of models best fits the data. For example, we may wish to know whether two particular regions are connected to one another based on the data. This can be achieved by comparing two models, one of which allows the connection and one of which does not (i.e., that parameter is fixed at zero). The relative fit of the two models can then be compared, and if the fit of the model with the path is significantly better than the model without the path, then we conclude that the connection exists. It is sometimes argued that model comparison should only be performed when the absolute fit of the model is good, but simulations by Protzner & McIntosh (2006) suggest that it is possible to find reliable differences between models even when the absolute fit of the model to the data is relatively poor.

It is critical to note that a model with more parameters will almost always fit the data better than a model with fewer parameters. Thus, we cannot simply compare the goodness of fit of the two models. Instead, we must use a model comparison statistic that takes into account the number of parameters in the model, such as the Akaike Information Criterion (AIC) or Bayesian Information Criterion (BIC). In other cases, we may wish to make inferences about the values of specific parameters of the model, rather than making comparisons between different models (cf. Stephan et al., 2010). For example, we may wish to determine whether the connection between two regions is positive or negative. This can be done by examining the estimated path values in the selected model.

8.3.2.3 Complications using SEM with fMRI data

There are a number of potential problems with using SEM on fMRI data. First, the standard methods for testing of SEM model fit assume independence between observations, which is not true of fMRI data. However, it is possible to adjust the degrees of freedom in the chi-squared test so that they reflect the *effective degrees of freedom*, which reflects the number of independent observations given the temporal autocorrelation in the data (Bullmore et al., 2000).

Most SEM studies have used a priori anatomical models to specify a graph and then performed hypothesis testing on that graph. However, failure to reject the model (through a nonsignificant chi-squared test) does not establish that it is the correct model, only that there is not enough evidence to reject it. As previously noted, it would be preferable to search all possible models to find the best-fitting one, given that our anatomical priors offer relatively weak starting points for building models of functional connectivity. For all but the smallest networks, exhaustively testing all possible models becomes computationally intractable, so search methods become necessary. The most common approach used in the SEM literature is a *greedy* search technique, in which one starts with a model with no connections and repeatedly adds the one connection that would most increase the model fit. This uses a technique called *Lagrangian multipliers* (Bullmore et al., 2000), also known in the SEM literature as *modification indices*. Unfortunately, it has been shown that this approach to network detection is unreliable because it tends to find local minima rather than the globally best network (Spirtes et al., 2000). The search methods described in the following section are known to outperform this approach.

Because SEM models are usually employed for fMRI analysis, another more fundamental problem is that the model is meant to identify causal relations between neuronal signals, but these must be estimated based on indirect and noisy BOLD MRI measurements (Penny et al., 2004). It can be shown (Ramsey et al., 2010) that when causal inferences about latent variables are based on indirect measurements, independent noise in the measurements will result in the identification of spurious relationships between some variables. In addition, the transformation from latent neuronal signals to observed hemodynamic signals is complex and nonlinear; even though such a relation could be accommodated with SEM, it is more naturally accommodated within approaches such as dynamic causal modeling (Section 8.3.4) that directly estimate the hemodynamic response function to estimate causal relations between neuronal elements.

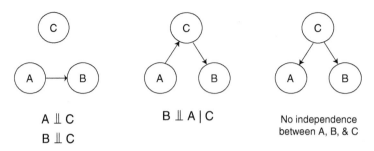

$A \perp\!\!\!\perp C$
$B \perp\!\!\!\perp C$

$B \perp\!\!\!\perp A \mid C$

No independence
between A, B, & C

Figure 8.9.　Each of the graphical models from Figure 8.1 implies a different set of conditional independence relations between the three nodes. Independence is denoted by $\perp\!\!\!\perp$, such that $B \perp\!\!\!\perp A \mid C$ means "B is independent of A after conditioning on C."

8.3.3 Graphical causal models

Another way to characterize the causal structure of a dataset has been developed in the context of graphical causal models (Spirtes et al., 2000; Shipley, 2000; Pearl, 2000). This approach is based on the idea that the causal relations in a graph have implications regarding the conditional independence relations between different sets of variables in the graph. Conditional independence means that two variables are independent when conditioned on some other variable(s) and Figure 8.9 illustrates examples of conditional independence based on the graphs from Figure 8.1. This idea will be familiar from the context of regression, where conditioning on a third variable is equivalent to including it as a covariate in the statistical model. If two variables are correlated via a third variable, then including that third variable as a regressor should remove the correlation, thus rendering the variables independent.

By determining the conditional independence relations that exist between a set of variables, it is possible to determine the graph or graphs that describe the causal relations that are implied by the pattern of conditional independence (Pearl, 2000; Spirtes et al., 2000). A set of methods developed in the field of machine learning over the last 20 years has provided the ability to efficiently search for such graphical structures.

A number of search algorithms exist for graph search, many of which are implemented in the freely available TETRAD software (see link on the book Web site). They differ primarily in the kinds of graphs that they are able to find (e.g., with or without cycles, with or without latent variables), and in their assumptions regarding the data (e.g., continuous vs. discrete, normally distributed versus nonnormal). A detailed description of these methods is outside the scope of this book; see Spirtes et al. (2000) and the TETRAD software manual for more details. Figure 8.10 shows an example of results using this software. Once the optimal graph(s) have been identified using these graph search methods, then they can be used as a basis for other kinds of effective connectivity models, such as SEM or dynamic causal models.

A: TETRAD (greedy equivalence search)

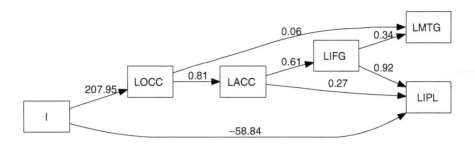

B: SEM (using modification indices)

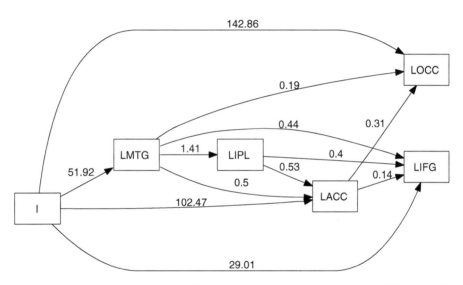

Figure 8.10. A comparison of the best-fitting models estimated using TETRAD IV and modification indices with structural equation modeling, using the example dataset. The data were timecourses from single voxels in five regions (LOCC: left occipital, LMTG: left middle temporal, LIPL: left inferior parietal, LACC: left anterior cingulate, LIFG: left inferior frontal), as well as an exogenous input representing the task convolved with a hemodynamic response. For the TETRAD example, the greedy equivalence search (GES) algorithm was used to search for the best-fitting graph, starting with the knowledge that the input was connected to LOCC. For the SEM example, a greedy search technique was applied as described by using the SEM function in R; starting with a basic model in which the input connected to LOCC, at each stage the edge that increased the model fit most greatly (as measured by modification indices) was added, until the chi-squared test for lack of model fit was no longer significant. The fit of the resulting networks was better for the TETRAD model (BIC = -27) than for the SEM model (BIC = -10).

One particular challenge to the use of search methods such as graphical causal modeling is to combine data across multiple subjects. Although it might seem most obvious to simply combine the data across subjects into a single search, or average the data across subjects, each of these has the potential to obtain incorrect results. As mentioned previously, the independence relations between variables that exist in a combined dataset may not reflect the relations that exist for any of the individuals. To address this issue, Ramsey et al. (2010) developed a method called IMaGES (independent multiply assessed greedy equivalence search), which performs a search across multiple subjects, even if those subjects do not share all of the same variables (e.g., if one subject has no significant signal within a particular ROI). This method, which is also available in the TETRAD software package, searches for the best-fitting graph structure, looking separately at each subject in each step of the search, and then combining the fit across subjects in order to find the model that fits best across the entire group.

8.3.4 Dynamic causal modeling

Whereas SEM and graphical causal models are very general methods that are applicable to many different kinds of data, dynamic causal modeling (DCM) (Friston et al., 2003) is a method developed specifically for the modeling of causal relations in neuroimaging data (fMRI and EEG/MEG). DCM attempts to infer the dynamics of the underlying neuronal systems from the observed fMRI signal. A DCM for fMRI is composed of two parts: A model of the *neurodynamics* (i.e., the underlying neuronal activity) and a model of the *hemodynamics* (i.e., the blood flow response induced by the neurodynamics).

The neurodynamic model in DCM is a differential equation (Penny et al., 2004):

$$\dot{z}_t = \left(A + \sum_{j=1}^{J} u_t(j) B^j \right) z_t + C u_t$$

where t indexes time, $\dot{z}_t$ is the derivative of neuronal activity in time, $u_t(j)$ is the jth of J extrinsic inputs at time t, and A, B^j, and C are *connectivity matrices*:

- A is the matrix of *intrinsic connections*, which specifies which regions are connected to one another and whether those connections are unidirectional or bidirectional.
- C is the matrix of *input connections*, which specifies which regions are affected by which extrinsic inputs u_j (e.g., stimuli or instructions).
- B^j are the *modulatory connections*, which specify how the intrinsic connections in A are changed by each of the u_j inputs.

DCM is often referred to as a *bilinear* model because it involves the interaction of two linear effects; however, the DCM model has also been extended to nonlinear cases in which connections are modulated by a third region (Stephan et al., 2008). The hemodynamic model in DCM is a version of the *balloon-windkessel model*

(Buxton et al., 1998; Mandeville et al., 1999), which models the relation between neuronal activity and changes in blood flow, blood volume, and blood oxygenation that result in the measured fMRI signal. These two models are combined in DCM to form a *generative model* of the fMRI signal, and given this model it is possible to simultaneously estimate the parameters of the neurodynamic model (i.e., the A, B^j, and C matrices) and hemodynamic model from fMRI data using Bayesian inference. The details of this estimation are quite complicated, and the interested reader should consult (Friston et al., 2003; Penny et al., 2004; Stephan et al., 2007) for more details.

Once the model parameters have been estimated, one can test hypotheses regarding specific connections or models. There are two classes of inference that are commonly made using DCM; a full explication of the DCM approach is provided by Stephan et al. (2010), and the interested reader is referred to that paper for very useful guidance regarding the use of DCM. Inference on the *model space* involves comparison of a set of DCMs in order to identify the model that best fits the observed data. For example, one might wish to know whether a model with a full set of modulatory connections fits the data better than models that are missing various ones of those connections. This employs model selection techniques, which take into account the complexity of the model in addition to its fit to the data. Inference on the *model parameters* involves the estimation of parameters for a particular model or for all of a set of models. For example, one might wish to know whether a specific modulatory parameter differs between two subjects groups. This question can be addressed using random effects analyses of the parameters that are estimated for each individual.

Although DCM is very powerful, it has some important limitations. First, as with SEM, the validity of the results depends upon the anatomical models that are specified and the regions that are used for data extraction. Although it is possible to perform trial-and-error search using DCM, this is unlikely to span a large enough part of the model space to accurately find the globally best model. Instead, one may consider using the graphical search techniques outlined earlier to construct a set of plausible candidate models, and then using DCM to test specific hypotheses about those models. Second, the current implmentation of DCM is limited to models with relatively few regions (due to memory limitations in MATLAB), though this may be alleviated by the use of 64-bit systems. Finally, recent work has shown that whereas DCM is highly reliable in model selection (e.g., across runs for the same individual), the exact parameter estimates can be relatively unreliable in cases where there are correlations between different parameter values (Rowe et al., 2010). Thus, analyses that rely upon the exact parameter values should be used with caution.

8.3.4.1 Using DCM

We fit the DCM model to the same data used in the previous examples in this chapter, using the same five ROIs as in Figure 8.10. The model of connectivity for DCM was based on the output from the TETRAD graph search. We first compared three different models. Model 1 allowed modulation of all connections by the task.

Model 2 had the same intrinsic connectivity but did not allow any modulation of intrinsic connections by the task. Model 3 was a "straw man" model that did not allow any intrinsic connections. Model comparison between these three models showed that Model 1 was the most likely, with a posterior probability of .995. As expected, comparison of Model 2 to Model 3 also showed that Model 2 was preferred, with a posterior probability approaching 1.

8.3.5 Granger causality

Granger causality is a method originally developed for the analysis of economic data, which models causality by examining the relation in time between variables. Granger causality is based on the notion that causes always precede effects in time. It is often framed in terms of a *multivariate autoregressive* (or MAR) model, where the values of a set of variables at some time t are modeled as a function of their values at earlier points in time. Given two variables X and Y, we say that X "Granger-causes" Y if the value of Y at time t is better predicted by the values of X and Y at time $t - 1$ than by the value of Y at time $t - 1$ alone. Granger causality has been applied in a whole-brain manner, known as *Granger causality mapping* (or GCM), whereby timecourse in a seed voxel is compared to all other voxels in the brain and Granger causality is computed for each voxel (Roebroeck et al., 2005).

Granger causality (and especially GCM) is a seemingly appealing alternative to other forms of effective connectivity modeling because it provides a way to examine whole-brain effective connectivity without the need for specifying an anatomical network, as is required for DCM and SEM. However, Granger causality analysis with fMRI data is problematic due to the temporal characteristics of fMRI data. First, since Granger causality relies upon the relative activity of regions in time, it is critical that the effects of slice timing be first accounted for; the differences in relative timing of acquisition across slices are likely to be much larger than the relative timing effects due to neural processing. Second, Granger causality assumes that the hemodynamic response is similar in its timing characteristics across the brain. However, this is known to be false (Miezin et al., 2000), and these differences in the timing of hemodynamic responses across brain regions will be manifest as spurious causes in a Granger causality analysis. In fact, it has been shown by David et al. (2008), using simultaneous electrophysiological recordings and fMRI, that Granger causality on fMRI timeseries does not accurately extract causal influences; on the other hand, when the timeseries were deconvolved to obtain estimates of the neuronal signal (using the hemodynamic model from DCM along with electrophysiological recordings), then Granger causality was able to correctly extract the causal relations that were observed in the electrophysiological data. Third, it is a known problem for Granger causality when the data are sampled at a rate slower than the causal process (as occurs when fMRI data are sampled on the order of seconds, when neuronal interactions occur on the order of milliseconds) (Ramsey et al., 2010; Swanson

& Granger, 1996). The proposed solution to this problem by Swanson & Granger (1996) is to obtain the residuals from a timeseries analysis and then to apply the graphical causal model search procedures described earlier (cf. Ramsey et al., 2010). Future developments may provide Granger causality methods that are more appropriate to fMRI data, but for the moment we discourage the use of Granger causality analysis with fMRI data.

8.4 Network analysis and graph theory

Another approach to modeling connectivity in fMRI data comes from a seemingly very different field: the study of social networks. Sociologists have long been interested in the so-called "six degrees of separation" phenomenon, whereby nearly everyone can find a path of friends to anyone else in the world in six or fewer steps. In the 1990s, a group of physicists began analyzing complex networks (such as the World Wide Web and the brain) and in doing so developed a new set of models for understanding the structure of a broad range of complex networks. A lively introduction to this area can be found in Watts (2003); a more detailed review can be found in Newman (2003), and an annotated collection of the classic papers in the area is found in Newman et al. (2006).

8.4.1 Small world networks

One of the fundamental contributions of network modeling has been the discovery and formal characterization of a kind of network, known as a *small world network*, which appears to be ubiquitous in complex systems. Small world networks have been discovered everywhere from the World Wide Web to the nervous system of the nematode *C. elegans* to the co-actor networks in films (made famous by the "Six Degrees of Kevin Bacon" game). Before describing a small world network, we first introduce a few important concepts from graph theory. A network is composed of a set of *nodes*, which are connected by links (known as *edges*). The *degree* of a node is the number of edges that it has. Now, let us first imagine a network where edges are placed randomly between nodes (known as a *random network*). If we examine the distribution of degree values (that is, the distribution of how connected each node is), we will see that it decreases exponentially, such that the number of heavily connected nodes is vanishingly small. However, when researchers started to examine complex networks such as the World Wide Web using these methods, they found that the degree distributions instead showed a long tail, such that there were more highly connected nodes than one would expect randomly. Networks with such degree distributions have small world characteristics, which means that the average distance between two nodes is less than one would expect in a randomly connected graph of the same size and mean degree. There is growing evidence that brain structure and function can both be characterized in terms of small world networks (Stephan et al., 2000; Bassett & Bullmore, 2006; Sporns et al., 2004), and analyses of network interactions in fMRI data have already provided important new insights. For example, analyses of resting state fMRI data across development have shown that the interactions between regions change over development in ways that are not obvious from the analysis of activation alone (Fair et al., 2007). Although it would be possible to apply network analysis methods to task-related fMRI data, it has generally been applied to resting-state data, which we will focus on here. An example resting state dataset is available from the book Web site.

8.4.2 Modeling networks with resting-state fMRI data

After properly preprocessing the data, the steps for network modeling with resting-state fMRI data are as follows:

1. *Extract data.* Network analyses vary in the number of nodes included in the analysis, but it is generally advisable to keep it as small as possible in order to optimize the analysis, as computations on more than a few thousand nodes become computationally very intensive. Often, signal is extracted from a limited number of regions of interest. For example, Fair et al. (2009) extracted data from 34 regions, which were based on previous studies. The preprocessed data from each of these regions is extracted and combined in an N (timepoints) $\times$ P (regions) matrix.

2. *Compute network adjacency.* Using the data extracted in step 2, we next compute a measure that indexes the strength of the relation between signals at each node in the network. The most common measure of adjacency is the Pearson correlation coefficient (r). The adjacency matrix is generally thresholded at some relatively liberal value (e.g., $r > 0.1$) in order to exclude edges that reflect noise. Another adjacency measure, known as topological overlap (Ravasz et al., 2002), computes the degree to which two nodes are highly correlated with the same other nodes (i.e., whether they are in the same correlational "neighborhood"). This measure may be more robust than simple correlation (Zhang & Horvath, 2005). For any adjacency measure, one must decide whether to use signed or unsigned (absolute) values, which reflects the nature of the question being asked (i.e., are negative correlations between nodes interesting?). After thresholding the adjacency matrix, this step results in a $P \times P$ matrix with binary entries specifying the presence or absence of a link between nodes.

3. *Characterize the network.* Having estimated the network from the adjacency measures, one can then characterize various aspects of the network, such as the average path length, clustering coefficient, or modularity measures. These measures may be useful in providing a general characterization of the topology of the network, such as the degree to which it exhibits a small world topology. There are a number of toolboxes available for performing these analyses in MATLAB, R, python, and other languages; links can be found on at the book Web site.

4. *Visualize the network.* Visualizing the network is the best way to apprehend its organization. An example is shown in Figure 8.11. It should be noted that there

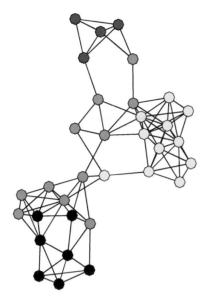

Figure 8.11. A example of a network obtained from analysis of resting state data. The data were obtained from the BIRN data repository and preprocessed as outlined in Section 8.4.3, followed by extraction of signal from the 34 nodes specified by Fair et al. (2009). The nodes are colored according to their involvement in each of the four network outlined by Fair et al. (2009): yellow, frontoparietal; black, cingulo-opercular; red, default mode; blue, cerebellar. The correlation matrix was thresholded in order to retain the highest 20% of connections between nodes. The data were visualized using the Kamada-Kawai spring-embedding algorithm, as implemented in the SNA package for R.

network visualization is as much art as science, and there are many different algorithms for graphical layout of a network. One should ensure that any conclusions based on the visualization are robust to different choices of visualization methods. In addition to static methods, there are also available tools such as SONIA (Moody et al., 2005) that allow animation of changes in network structure (e.g., as might occur across learning or development).

8.4.3 Preprocessing for connectivity analysis

An important consideration when carrying out connectivity analysis is that artifacts, such as head motion, may cause spurious connections between regions of the brain. To avoid such false positive connections, these trends can be removed from the data prior to analyzing connectivity between regions. In the case of resting state data, the correlations that are of interest are driven by low-frequency trends in the data, which is also where many of the noise signals (aliased and otherwise) typically seen in fMRI data tend to be. In order to improve the quality of the connectivity analysis, removal of nuisance trends from the data is necessary. For resting state fMRI, the typical nuisance trends considered for removal from the data include the six motion parameters resulting from rigid body motion correction (along with their first derivatives), the average signal from the white matter, ventricular signal, global mean, and physiologic signals such as the heart rate and respiration (Cohen et al., 2008; Birn et al., 2006; Fox et al., 2005). There is some debate on whether the global mean should or should not be removed from the data. Interestingly, including the global signal in standard *task*-based fMRI data analysis is typically discouraged, since it has been shown to reduce activation when there is widespread activation corresponding to a task, and false negative activations can also result (Aguirre et al., 1998; Junghofer et al., 2005; Gavrilescu et al., 2002). In the case of resting state fMRI, the motivation for including the global mean is that the global signal will contain information on nonneuronal signal artifacts, such as components related to motion and respiration. Some work has indicated that treating the global signal as a nuisance in resting-state fMRI data analysis may induce false negative correlations (Murphy et al., 2009; Weissenbacher et al., 2009; Cole et al., 2010), but there is still a debate on whether these negative correlations are mathematical epiphenomena or reflect meaningful aspects of brain function. In general, negative correlations found when modeling the global signal should be interpreted carefully, and since the bias is toward negative correlations, significant positive correlations are not likely to be false positives.

Depending on what type of connectivity analysis is conducted, removal of the nuisance signal is done in different ways. In the case of seed-based connectivity analyses, one would want the analysis to reflect partial correlation coefficients between the seed voxel and all other target voxels. This is achieved by running a regression analysis with each BOLD time series as the dependent variable, modeling the nuisance parameters as independent variables as well as carrying out other operations such as smoothing, high-pass filtering, and low-pass filtering. Then the residuals resulting from this analysis would be used to calculate Pearson correlation coefficients in the seed-based connectivity analysis. After properly reducing the degrees of freedom by the number of nuisance parameters that were adjusted for, the inferences on these correlations correspond to tests of the partial correlation coefficients. Note that prewhitening, although standard with task-based fMRI data analysis, would not be used with resting state fMRI, as it might filter out important low-frequency fluctuations that drive the resting state network (Shmuel & Leopold, 2008).

In the case of a PPI analysis, the nuisance trends should also be removed from the data prior to the creation of the PPI regressor. If it weren't for the modulation that is carried out when creating the PPI regressor, the nuisance trends could simply be added to the model with the PPI regressor. Suppose both the target voxel and the seed voxel/region exhibit two positive spikes during two trials, one of each trial type to be contrasted in the PPI regressor. For the PPI regressor, in one case the spike will remain positive for one task, but due to the modulation of the PPI regressor, the other spike will be negative. Although the motion parameter can be added to the model, it may not model the spikes very well, since they may be in different directions in the PPI regressor. The solution is to remove all nuisance trends from the data prior to creation of the seed time series and creation of the PPI regressor. This would be accomplished as previously described in the case of resting-state data. Of course, inferences should account for the additional degrees of freedom that were used in the nuisance model.

Lastly, for independent component analysis, it is not necessary to model nuisance parameters from the data, since the nuisance components will automatically be separated from the resting-state network components. The challenge is separating out these two groups of components, although an approach for identifying resting state network components based on how well they match the default mode network (Greicius & Menon, 2004; Greicius et al., 2007).

Multivoxel pattern analysis and machine learning

9.1 Introduction to pattern classification

The statistical methods discussed in the book so far have had the common feature of trying to best characterize the dataset at hand. For example, when we apply the general linear model to a dataset, we use methods that determine the model parameters that best describe that dataset (where "best" means "with the lowest mean squared difference between the observed and fitted data points"). The field known variously as *machine learning*, *statistical learning*, or *pattern recognition* takes a different approach to modeling data. Instead of finding the model parameters that best characterize the observed data, machine learning methods attempt to find the model parameters that allow the most accurate prediction for new observations. The fact that these are not always the same is one of the most fundamental intuitions that underlies this approach.

The field of machine learning is enormous and continually growing, and we can only skim the surface of these methods in this chapter. At points we will assume that the reader has some familiarity with the basic concepts of machine learning. For readers who want to learn more, there are several good textbooks on machine learning methods, including Alpaydin (2004), Bishop (2006), Duda et al. (2001), and Hastie et al. (2001). With regard to the specific application of machine learning methods to fMRI, often referred to as *multivoxel pattern analysis* or *MVPA*, excellent reviews include Haynes & Rees (2006), Norman et al. (2006), and O'Toole et al. (2007) Links to software packages for machine learning analysis can be found on the book Web site.

9.1.1 An overview of the machine learning approach

The goal of machine learning is to maximize the ability to make predictions about data that have not yet been observed; that is, we wish to *generalize* from the observed data to yet-unseen data. For example, we may wish to use fMRI data to predict which of two drugs will more effectively treat a new psychiatric patient or to decode the kind of mental process that an individual is engaged in. When the prediction is one of a set of discrete categories, we refer to it as *classification*, whereas when it is a continuous value we refer to it as *regression*; since nearly all applications to fMRI have used classification rather than regression, we will refer generally to classification and regression machines as *classifiers*.

9.1.1.1 Features, observations, and the "curse of dimensionality"

In machine learning, we aim to learn the relation between a set of observed features (in our case, the intensity of voxels) and some outcome variable (e.g., mental state or psychiatric diagnosis) over some set of observations (usually either individual trials or individual subjects). However, in fMRI (as in many other modern data analysis problems), the number of features (usually more than 50,000) is many times greater than the number of observations (20–100). This makes it impossible to fit a standard GLM model to the data using standard techniques, since the number of features in a GLM must be less than the number of observations to estimate a unique set of parameters. The large number of dimensions also poses a more fundamental problem in modeling. To adequately model a dataset, we need to measure systematically across the range of each variable being measured. For example, if we want to examine the relation between height and weight, we need to sample individuals whose height varies across the entire range of the population. However, as we add dimensions, the number of samples that are required to cover the range of all dimensions grows exponentially; this problem is known as the "curse of dimensionality" (Bellman, 1961).

The field of machine learning is largely concerned with developing methods to deal with this curse. One way to do so is to reduce the number of dimensions. For example, if there is redundant information across many dimensions, then one can use *dimensionality reduction* techniques such as principal components analysis or independent components analysis to identify a smaller set of alternative dimensions that give rise to the data. Another way to address the curse is to assume that the signal is sparse in the data, and focus on a small number of features. This can be done either by using a classifier that is designed to find sparse solutions, or through the use of *feature selection* techniques that reduce the number of features being examined.

9.1.1.2 Overfitting

One might think that the model that fits the observed data best would be most likely to also predict new outcomes most accurately, but it is easy to see that this is not the case (see Figure 9.1). A more complex model (i.e., a model with more parameters) will always fit the training data more accurately; in the limit, if there are as many parameters as there are data points, then the data can be fit perfectly. However, if the actual function relating these variables is less complex (e.g., a linear or quadratic function), then using a more complex model will result in *overfitting*, in which the model fit is driven largely by noise in the training data. This results in a better fit for the training data but worse generalization to the test data, as show in Figure 9.1.

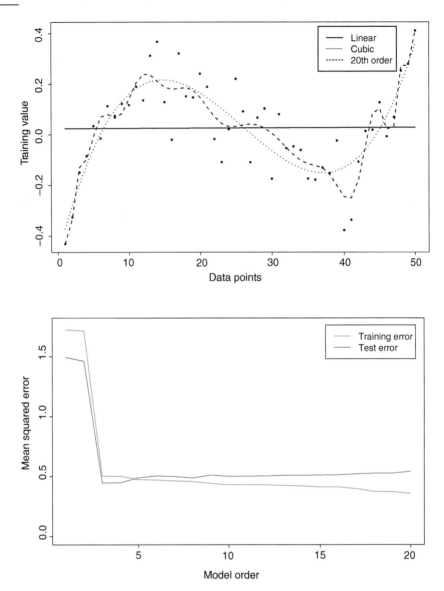

Figure 9.1.   An example of overfitting. The left panel shows a set of data points created by adding random
Gaussian noise to a cubic function. The data were then fitted using three different models: A
linear model (solid line), the correct cubic model (dotted line), and a 20th-order polynomial
model (dashed line). The cubic model clearly fits the response. The linear model underfits the
data, whereas the 20th-order model overfits the data, adapting its response to noise present
in many of the individual data points. The right panel shows the fit of the model to the training
data and to a test dataset generated using the same function with independent noise values.
Whereas increasing the model order always increases the fit to the training data, the fit of the
model to the test data actually decreases as the model order increases beyond the true value
of 3, reflecting overfitting to the training data.

9.2 Applying classifiers to fMRI data

The process of applying a classifier to fMRI data (often referred to as multivoxel pattern analysis or MVPA) follows four steps:

- *Data extraction*: Extract the data that will be used to train and test the classifier.
- *Feature selection*: Select which features will be included in the analysis.
- *Training and testing*: Train the classifier on the dataset and determine its accuracy at out-of-sample generalization.
- *Classifier characterization*: Determine which features are most important for classification accuracy.

9.3 Data extraction

The data that are extracted from the fMRI timeseries depend upon the nature of the classification problem. For classification of different events for a particular individual (which we will call *within-subject* classification), the challenge is to extract the features that best reflect the activity evoked by each event. This is relatively easy for blocked designs because there are sets of timepoints that can be uniquely attributed to each particular condition. One can either include all of the timepoints within a block, or use some summary of the timepoints such as the mean or the beta of a GLM model for the block. For event-related designs with relatively long intertrial intervals (greater than about 10 seconds), we can extract the signal evoked on each event with relatively little contamination due to other events; one can either use the beta-series correlation model discussed in Section 8.2.3, or use a simpler approach in which one simply takes the single timepoint that occurs 4–6 seconds after the event, which should capture the peak of the hemodynamic response. For rapid event-related designs, the overlap between different events makes the data extraction problem much more difficult. One alternative method applicable to both slow and rapid event-related designs is to use a beta-series approach (Section 8.2.3). However, for rapid designs the closeness of the events in time may result in substantial correlations in the design matrix that will cause highly variable estimates. It is possible to use ridge regression in order to address this problem (Rizk-Jackson et al., 2008) but the sensitivity of this approach will almost certainly be low.

Another alternative is to enter the entire timecourse of each trial into the classifier, which is known as a *spatiotemporal classifier* (Mourão-Miranda et al., 2007). In this case, the classifier will determine which timepoints contain relevant information. This approach has the benefit of not assuming any particular shape for the hemodynamic response and thus may be more sensitive if the response differs from the canonical shape. However, it also greatly increases the number of features and could make it more difficult for some classifiers to learn. We would generally recommend that researchers who are interested in applying machine learning methods should use either blocked designs or relatively slow event-related designs to mitigate the severe feature extraction problems that arise with rapid event-related designs.

Another alternative is to forego trial-by-trial classification and instead classify between summary statistic maps estimated for separate portions of the data (e.g., separate runs) (e.g., Haxby et al., 2001; Haynes et al., 2007) This eliminates the problems with estimation of trial-by-trial responses, but it does slightly change the conclusions that one can draw from the results; rather than implying that one can accurately decode individual trials, it instead provides a more general measure of how much information is present regarding the distinction that is being classified. A similar approach can be used for studies that attempt to classify across individuals; in this case, it is most common to use some form of spatially normalized summary map for each individual, such as a parameter estimate map or t/Z-statistic map. There may be some utility in using statistical maps rather than parameter estimate maps because they have the same scaling across voxels.

9.4 Feature selection

Having extracted the relevant data from the fMRI timeseries, the next step is to determine which features (voxels) to include in the classifier analysis. There are two possible layers of feature selection. First, we can identify a set of voxels in a way that does not involve any knowledge of the outcome variable, either using a priori anatomical knowledge or features of the data that are unrelated to the outcome variable. Second, we can use the classifier to identify which voxels are most useful for classification, and use just those features in the analysis. The former is discussed here; the latter, in Section 9.5.

Most simply, one can just include the data from the entire brain (Poldrack et al., 2009; Hanson & Halchenko, 2008). Depending upon the voxel size, this can be up to 300,000 features, which is beyond the limits of some classifiers (e.g., neural networks) and stretches the limits of many others. Support vector machines are generally the classifier of choice for this kind of analysis, as they perform well even with very large numbers of features (but still sometimes benefit from further feature selection). The whole-brain approach is most appropriate when the question of interest is whether there is information in the brain relevant to some particular functional distinction, without regard to where that information is found (though it is possible to obtain localization for some whole-brain classifiers using the classifier characterization methods to be discussed in Section 9.6).

It is also possible to limit the analysis to particular voxels using a priori regions of interest. Various strategies for specification of ROIs are discussed in Section 10.4.2 and include the use of individualized anatomical labels or population-based anatomical atlases as well as independent functional localizers. This strategy can be particularly useful when the goal is to identify the relative importance of particular anatomically or functionally defined region in a specific function or to focus on a particular region of prior interest. It is important to ensure that the selection of ROI is not based on any knowledge of the results from the analysis, since this could bias the resulting generalization estimates.

Beyond anatomically driven feature selection, it is also possible to perform unsupervised feature selection using characteristics of the individual features that are unrelated to the outcome variable. For example, we might choose those features that have the highest variance across observations, under the assumption that they are likely to carry more information about differences between observations than would less-variable features.

9.5 Training and testing the classifier

Once we have preprocessed the data, the next step is to train the classifier and assess its generalization performance (by comparing its predictions to the known true values of the outcome variable). To accurately assess the performance of the classifier in generalization to new data, it is critical that we use separate datasets to train and test the classifier (see Box 9.5.2). The simplest way to do this would be to collect two datasets, using one to train the classifier and the other to test it. However, this would be inefficient, since we would have to collect twice the number of observations that we would otherwise collect. In addition, the results would be rather variable, since they would depend upon which observations randomly appear in the study and test samples. Fortunately, there are much more effective ways to assess generalization ability, which take advantage of the fact that we can use the same data for training and testing if we do so in separate training–testing iterations. This procedure goes by the name of *cross-validation*; it is often referred to as *k-fold cross-validation* reflecting the fact that the data are broken into k blocks of observations, and the classifier is trained on all blocks but one, then tested on the left-out block, which is then repeated for all blocks. If k is equal to the number of observations, then this is called *leave-one-out* cross-validation. Leave-one-out cross-validation is relatively costly in terms of computation (since the classifier has to be fit for each left-out observation) but will provide an unbiased measure of test accuracy, whereas cross-validation with larger k may sometimes be biased; ten-fold cross-validation appears to be a good compromise (Hastie et al., 2009).

9.5.1 Feature selection/elimination

It is common to use feature selection within the cross-validation cycle to reduce the number of features by excluding noninformative features (which add noise but no signal). For example, we can perform a statistical test to determine whether each voxel shows a statistically significant difference between conditions. A more sophisticated approach is known as *recursive feature elimination* (Guyon et al., 2002), in which

Box 9.5.2 The importance of separate training and test data

The goal of any classifier analysis is an accurate assessment of generalization, that is, performance on a test dataset that is completely separate from the data used to train the classifier. However, information about the test set can be insidious, and any contamination of the training data with the test data will result in an overestimate of generalization performance. It is thus extremely important to ensure that the training procedure does not involve any "peeking" at the test data. One good clue that contamination has occurred is when one sees classifier performance that is *too good*; if generalization performance on a test set is at 99% accuracy, it is very likely that some contamination has occurred.

A good general strategy for identifying contamination is to execute the entire processing stream using a dataset where the relationship between the features and outcomes has been broken (e.g., by randomly reassigning the outcomes across observations). This requires the assumption of exchangeability (Nichols & Holmes, 2002) (see Section 7.3.1.4), so it is important to make sure that the units of reassignment are exchangeable under the null hypothesis. It is useful to have a processing stream that is completely automated, so that this can be run many times and the average accuracy can be computed. Because the average accuracy should be identical to chance in this situation, any bias should be evident.

As an example, let's say that we wish to classify which of two classes of stimuli is present based on signal from a set of voxels. (A simulation of this analysis is available on the book Web site.) We would like to limit our analysis only to voxels that are likely to show an effect of the stimulus class, to reduce the impact of noise on our analysis, which can be determined using a standard univariate statistical test at each voxel. As a simple procedure, let's take half of the data as our training data and the other half as the test data. We could perform the univariate test over the entire dataset (training + test halves), taking the voxels that show the greatest difference between classes in that dataset. Alternatively, we could perform the same feature selection using only the data from the training set. If we perform these analyses in a simulation where there is true signal present, we will see that both of them will show significant classification accuracy, but the procedure that includes the test data will show slightly higher generalization accuracy. The bias due to including test data in the feature selection procedure is even more evident when we simulate what happens when there is not actually any signal present. In this case, the procedure using only the training data to select features exhibits accuracy of 50%, as one would expect when there is no signal present. However, the procedure using both training and test data to select features shows accuracy above chance; for example, if there are 1,000 voxels and we choose the top 10 for inclusion in the analysis, the test accuracy will be around 75%, even though there is no signal actually present! The reason for this false accuracy is that the feature

> **Box 9.5.2** (*Continued*)
>
> selection procedure found those voxels that just happened to have differences in signal between the classes (due to random noise) in both the training and test phases. This analysis highlights the utility and importance of simulating one's entire analysis stream using noise data.

the classifier is iteratively fit and at each step a certain number or proportion of the least informative features is removed. Such approaches can in some cases be useful to increase classifier performance. It is critical that feature selection is performed on training data that are separate from the test set; if the test data are used in the feature selection step, then the test results are likely to be compromised (see Box 9.5.2).

Feature selection can also be accomplished using *dimensionality reduction* techniques to reduce the data to a smaller number of dimensions, which may nonetheless carry nearly all of the information present in the larger dataset (due to correlations among features). For example, the matrix decomposition methods discussed in Section 8.2.5, such as PCA and ICA, can be used for this purpose.

9.5.2 Classifiers for fMRI data

Before performing a classification analysis, it is necessary to choose which of the myriad available techniques one will use.

9.5.2.1 Linear vs. nonlinear classifiers

Classifiers vary in the kinds of statistical relations that they can detect. *Linear* classifiers can detect effects where it is possible to separate the data points associated with each class using a linear function; in two dimensions this is a line, whereas in high-dimensional spaces this will be a *hyperplane*. *Nonlinear* classifiers can detect effects that are defined by more complex functions. Figures 9.2 and 9.3 show examples of a range of classifiers (both linear and nonlinear) applied to classification problems that are linear and nonlinear, respectively.

The literature on fMRI classification has largely used linear classifiers, for several reasons. First, linear classifiers are generally the simplest to understand (though some nonlinear classifiers, such as quadratic discriminant analysis, are also quite simple). Second, linear classifiers are generally easier to characterize, as discussed in Section 9.6. Third, nonlinear classifiers have additional parameters that require optimization, and this generally requires an additional layer of cross-validation (since the parameter optimization must be independent of the test data). Despite this, there will clearly be some problems for which linear classifiers fail but nonlinear classifiers succeed, and it is important to include nonlinear classifiers in any relative assessment of classifier performance.

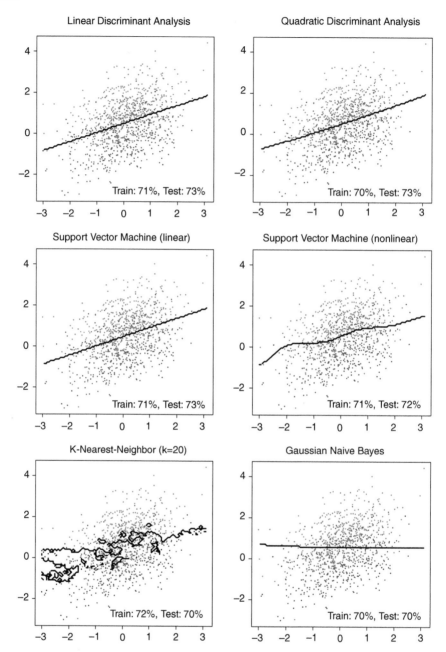

Figure 9.2.   Performance of a range of classifiers on a linear classification problem. The data for each were generated from a multivariate normal distribution, with a difference of 1.0 in the means between classes along the Y dimension. The red and blue dots are for observations from each class, respectively, and the black line in each figure reflect the category boundary estimated by each classifier. The training accuracy presented in each figure is for the data presented in the figure, whereas the test accuracy is for another dataset sampled from the same distribution. All of the classifiers perform very similarly, with slightly worse test performance of the nearest-neighbor classifier due to overfitting.

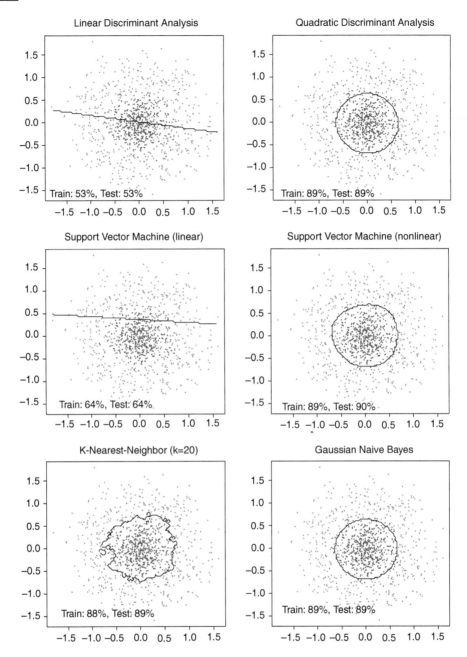

Figure 9.3.   Performance of a range of classifiers on a nonlinear classification problem. The data for each class were generated using a multivariate normal distribution transformed into a circle, with a difference in the radius of 1.0 between classes. In this case, the linear classifiers (LDA and linear SVM) perform relatively badly in comparison to the nonlinear classifiers, which are able to accurately detect the circular class boundary. The linear SVM performs somewhat above chance by capitalizing on the different distributions of the two classes, even though its boundary is not correct for this problem.

9.5.2.2 Computational limitations

Classifiers also vary in the size of the feature sets they can accommodate, and their efficiency at fitting large datasets. Some classifiers (such as support vector machines) can be implemented in such a way that very large datasets (e.g., several hundred thousand features) can be fit in a reasonable amount of time (e.g., 1–2 hours). Others, such as neural networks, are feasible with datasets up to about 5,000 to 10,000 features, at which point memory requirements become a limiting factor (depending upon the specific algorithm and implementation). In addition, fitting of these models can take a very long time. At the other end of the spectrum are classifiers, such as linear discriminant analysis, that require that the number of features is less than the number of observations; these methods are generally used in conjunction with some form of dimensionality reduction in order to address this limitation.

9.5.2.3 Tendency to overfit

Classifiers also vary in their tendency to overfit the data. Some classifiers, such as one-nearest-neighbor classifiers and simple neural network methods, are very likely to overfit the data, resulting in very good training performance but very bad generalization. However, most classification techniques use some form of *regularization* to prevent overfitting. Further, some techniques (such as support vector machines) are specifically designed to prevent overfitting.

9.5.3 Which classifier is best?

There is a large literature focused on the development of newer and better classifier techniques, and one often sees papers in the fMRI literature that report the application of a novel classifier technique to fMRI data, touting its performance in comparison to other methods. It is critical to realize, however, that although particular classifiers may work well for particular datasets or problems, no single method is superior across all datasets and classification problems. This can in fact be proven formally and is known as the *"no free lunch" theorem* in machine learning (Duda et al., 2001). Each particular classifier will perform well on datasets that are well-matched to its particular assumptions, whereas the same classifier could perform very badly on other datasets that are mismatched. It is thus important to test a range of classifiers to ensure that the results of any study are not limited by the nature of the particular classifier being studied. Using tools such as the PyMVPA toolbox or the R software package, it is possible to assess the performance of a large panel of classifiers on any dataset, which will likely provide the best guidance as to which classifier is most appropriate to the problem at hand. Again here, it is important that any such model selection is performed on data that are separate from the ultimate test data.

9.5.4 Assessing classifier accuracy

We often wish to determine whether the generalization accuracy of a classifier is better than would be expected by chance. A simple way to assess this is by comparing performance to that expected according to some null distribution under change (e.g., a binomial distribution for a two-alternative classification). However, if there is any bias in the classifier, this will be inaccurate; for example, if there are unequal numbers of observations in each class, this may introduce bias in the accuracy. A more accurate way to quantify performance versus chance is to use a resampling approach, in which the entire cross-validation procedure is performed multiple times with the class labels randomly reassigned each time (again under the assumption of exchangeability). The accuracy values for each run are stored, and their distribution provides an empirical null distribution against which the observed performance can be tested.

It is also important to examine accuracy separately for all classes of observations, rather than simply computing overall accuracy across all observations. One case in which the use of overall accuracy can be particularly problematic is when there are unequal numbers of observations in each class. Some classifiers will tend to simply assign all observations to the more common class; thus, if 80% of the observations fall into one class, then the classifier will perform at 80% accuracy, even though it has learned nothing except the fact that one class is more common than the other. One solution to this problem is to compute a balanced accuracy measure, which is the average accuracy for each class of stimuli. In addition, when class frequencies are unequal, it may be useful to employ a stratified cross-validation scheme, in which the proportion of class members is equated across each cross-validation fold (Kohavi, 1995). For regression models, it is also useful to balance the distribution of feature values across folds (Cohen et al., 2010); otherwise, differences in distributions across folds may result in systematically incorrect predictions on test data.

9.6 Characterizing the classifier

Having performed a classifier analysis and found that it performs well on the selected feature set, it is important to assess how the classifier achieves its performance. In general, this will involve characterizing the role that each feature plays in the classification.

Sensitivity maps.   One common procedure is to visualize the importance of each voxel for the classification, creating what are often called *sensitivity maps* or *importance maps*. The specific nature of this step will depend upon the kind of classifier that is used. For example, with neural networks, it is possible to map the weight structure of the network back onto the brain, providing an *importance map* that notes each voxel's contribution to the classification performance. With support vector machines, it is also possible to compute sensitivity maps based on the parameters assigned to each dimension. With any such maps, it is important to keep in mind that they reflect the sensitivity of the particular classifier that was chosen for the analysis, and that different classifiers may be sensitive to different features. In addition, sensitivity may not imply that the feature is important for generalization. Nonetheless, sensitivity maps are often useful for better understanding how the classifier achieves its performance.

It is also possible to assess the importance of features by examining the effect of disrupting them by adding noise. For example, Hanson et al. (2004) did this using a neural network classifier, adding noise to each input voxel and choosing those where noise affected performance by at least 30%. The exact nature of the noise is likely to be important, depending upon the classifier, so this approach is recommended only for users who have a very solid understanding of classifier behavior.

The searchlight procedure.   Another technique that has been used to characterize regional classifier performance is the *searchlight* (Kriegeskorte et al., 2006). In this method, a small sphere is placed with its center at each voxel, and the classifier is trained and tested using only voxels within that sphere; the test accuracy is then assigned to the center voxel. This provides a map showing which regions contain information relevant to classification. Searchlight maps are particularly useful because they can be used in a group analysis to find regions that show consistent classification accuracy across subjects. There are two potential difficulties with searchlight analyses. First, depending upon the speed of the particular classifier, the resolution of the data, and the choice of searchlight radius, running a searchlight at every voxel in the brain can result in very long computation times. Second, the choice of radius may affect the nature of the results; a very large searchlight will potentially integrate information across multiple functional regions, whereas a very small searchlight will integrate information over just a few voxels. The appropriate choice of searchlight radius depends upon the hypothesis that is being tested.

Once searchlight maps are obtained, it is necessary to threshold them in order to identify which regions show significant classification performance. For individual subjects, one common practice is to threshold the map using a binomial test. However, this approach can be problematic if there is any bias in the classifier, so it is best to use permutation testing as described earlier. For group analyses, the searchlight sensitivity maps can be submitted to a standard GLM analysis treating subjects as a random effect.

Visualizing, localizing, and reporting fMRI data

The dimensionality of fMRI data is so large that, in order to understand the data, it is necessary to use visualization tools that make it easier to see the larger patterns in the data. Parts of this chapter are adapted from Devlin & Poldrack (2007) and Poldrack (2007).

10.1 Visualizing activation data

It is most useful to visualize fMRI data using a tool that provides simultaneous viewing in all three canonical orientations at once (see Figure 10.1), which is available in all of the major analysis packages.

Because we wish to view the activation data overlaid on brain anatomy, it is necessary to choose an anatomical image to serve as an underlay. This anatomical image should be as faithful as possible to the functional image being overlaid. When viewing an individual participant's activation, the most accurate representation is obtained by overlaying the statistical maps onto that individual's own anatomical scan coregistered to the functional data. When viewing activation from a group analysis, the underlay should reflect the anatomical variability in the group as well as the smoothing that has been applied to the fMRI data. Overlaying the activation on the anatomical image from a single subject, or on a single-subject image, implies a degree of anatomical precision that is not actually present in the functional data. Instead, the activation should be visualized on an average structural image from the group coregistered to the functional data, preferably after applying the same amount of spatial smoothing as was applied to the functional data. Although this appears less precise due to the blurring of macroanatomical landmarks, it accurately reflects the imprecision in the functional data due to underlying anatomical variability and smoothing.

After choosing an appropriate underlay, it is then necessary to choose how to visualize the statistical map. Most commonly, the map is visualized after thresholding,

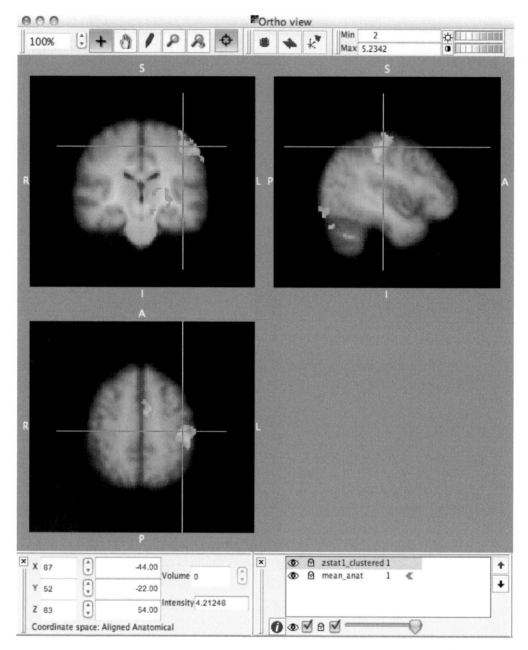

Figure 10.1. An example of group fMRI activation overlaid on orthogonal sections, viewed using FSLView. The underlay is the mean anatomical image from the group of subjects.

showing only those regions that exhibit significant activation at a particular threshold. For individual maps and exploratory group analyses, it is often useful to visualize the data at a relatively weak threshold (e.g., $p < .01$ uncorrected) in order to obtain a global view of the data. It can also be useful to visualize the data in an unthresholded

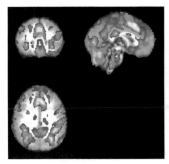 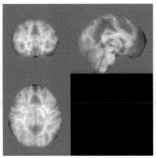 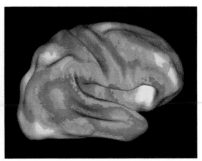

Figure 10.2. Various ways of viewing fMRI activation maps. Left panel: Standard thresholded activation maps, showing positive activation in red/yellow and negative activation in blue/green. Middle panel: True color map of the same data, showing positive signals in red and negative signals in blue, created using the mricron software package. Right panel: Rendering of the same data onto the cortical surface, using the CARET software package.

manner, using truecolor maps (see Figure 10.2). This gives a global impression of the nature of the statistical map and also provides a view of which regions are not represented in the statistical map due to dropout or artifacts, as well as showing both positive and negative effects. For inference, however, we always suggest using a corrected threshold.

Another way to view activation data is to project them onto the cortical surface, as shown in Figure 10.2. This can be a very useful way to visualize activation, as it provides a three-dimensional perspective that can be difficult to gain from anatomical slices alone. In addition, data can be registered by alignment of cortical surface features and then analyzed in surface space, which can sometimes provide better alignment across subjects than volume-based alignment (e.g., Desai et al., 2005). However, these methods often require substantial processing time and manual intervention to accurately reconstruct the cortical surface. Recently, a method has been developed that allows projection of individual or group functional activation onto a population-based surface atlas (Van Essen, 2005). This method, known as multifiducial mapping, maps the activation data from a group analysis onto the cortical surfaces of a group of (different) subjects and then averages those mappings, thus avoiding the bias that would result from mapping group data onto a single subject's surface. Although individual reconstruction will remain the gold standard for mapping activation data to the cortical surface, the multifiducial mapping technique (implemented in the CARET software package) provides a useful means for viewing projections of group activation data on a population-averaged cortical surface.

SPM includes two visualization tools that are often used but can result in mislocalization if used inappropriately. The first is the "glass brain" rendering that has been used since the early days of PET analysis (see Figure 10.3). This is a three-dimensional

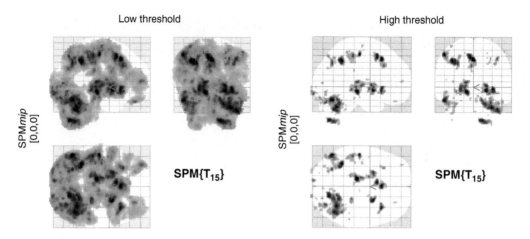

Figure 10.3. An example of SPM's glass brain visualization, showing maximum intensity projections along each axis. At a lower threhsold (shown the left panel), there are a relatively large number of regions active, which makes it relatively difficult to determine the location of activation. At a higher threshold (right panel), it becomes easier to identify the location of activated regions.

projection known as a "maximum intensity projection" as it reflects the strongest signal along each projection through the brain for the given axis. Using the glass brain figures to localize activation requires substantial practice, and even then it is difficult to be very precise. In addition, if large amounts of activation are present, as in the left panel of Figure 10.3, it can be difficult to differentiate activated regions.

The SPM "rendering" tool is often used to project activation onto the brain surface for visualization (see Figure 10.4). It is important to note, however, that this is not a proper rendering; rather, it is more similar to the maximum intensity projection used for the glass brain. Our recommendation for visualization of group activation on the cortical surface would be to project the data into cortical surface space, using CARET or FreeSurfer, which will lead to more precise localization.

10.2 Localizing activation

One of the most common questions on the mailing lists for fMRI analysis software packages is some variant of the following: "I've run an analysis and obtained an activation map. How can I determine what anatomical regions are activated?" As outlined by Devlin & Poldrack (2007), there are two approaches to this question. One (which we refer to as "black-box anatomy") is to use an automated tool to identify activation locations, which requires no knowledge of neuroanatomy. The alternative, which we strongly suggest, is to use knowledge of neuroanatomy along with a variety of atlases to determine which anatomical regions are activated.

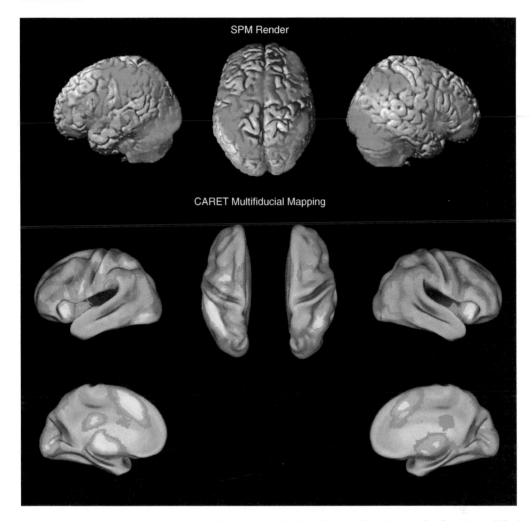

Figure 10.4. The top panel shows an activation map displayed using the SPM Render function, while the bottom section shows the same data rendered to the cortical surface using CARET's multifiducial mapping function. The CARET rendering provides substantially greater anatomical detail.

Having overlaid activation on the appropriate anatomical image, there are a number of neuroanatomical atlases available to assist in localization of activation, as well as some useful Web sites (listed on the book Web site).

10.2.1 The Talairach atlas

Probably the best known atlas for human brain anatomy is the one developed by Jean Talairach (Talairach, 1967; Talairach & Tournoux, 1988). However, as we argued in Devlin & Poldrack (2007), there are a number of reasons why we do not recommend using this atlas or the various automated tools derived from it. In short, we believe that localization based on the Talairach atlas is an alluringly easy but bad option. It is easy because the atlas has an overlaid coordinate system, which makes it trivial to identify an activated location. It is nonetheless a bad option because this provides a false sense of precision and accuracy, for a number of reasons:

1. The atlas is based on the single brain of a 60-year-old woman, and therefore is not representative of either the population as a whole nor any individuals.

2. Almost all major analysis packages use the templates based on the MNI305 atlas as their target for spatial normalization, which are population-based (and therefore representative) templates. An extra step is needed to convert coordinates into Talairach space, and this introduces additional registration error. Worse still, there is no consensus regarding how to perform this transformation (Brett et al., 2002; Carmack et al., 2004; Lancaster et al., 2007) and therefore the chosen method biases the results, introducing additional variation and therefore reducing accuracy.

3. The atlas is based on a single left hemisphere that was reflected to model the other hemisphere. However, there are well-known hemispheric asymmetries in normal individuals (e.g., location of Heschl's gyrus, length of precentral gyrus), such that assuming symmetry across hemispheres will result in additional inaccuracy.

4. The Talairach atlas is labeled with Brodmann's areas, but the precision of these labels is highly misleading. The labels were transferred manually from the Brodmann's map by Talairach, and even according to Talairach the mapping is uncertain (cf., Brett et al., 2002; Uylings et al., 2005).

For all of these reasons, the Talairach atlas is not a good choice. Likewise, we believe that automated coordinate-based labeling methods based on the Talairach atlas (such as the Talairach Daemon: Lancaster et al., 2000) are problematic. We believe that it is much better to take the nominally more difficult, but far more accurate, route of using an anatomical atlas rather than one based on coordinates.

10.2.2 Anatomical atlases

One atlas that we find particularly useful is the Duvernoy atlas (Duvernoy & Bourgouin, 1999), which presents MRI images in all three canonical planes as well as photographs of matching brain slices. The lack of a coordinate system in the atlas forces one to localize not by coordinates but in terms of relevant macroanatomical landmarks. In addition to Duvernoy (which has unfortunately gone out of print), there are several other atlases that can also be useful (e.g., Mai et al., 2004; Woolsey et al., 2008), and there are specialty atlases for specific brain regions such as cerebellum (Schmahmann, 2000), hippocampus (Duvernoy, 2005), subcortical structures (Lucerna et al., 2004), and white matter tracts (Mori et al., 2004). The highly skilled neuroanatomist may be able to accurately label most structures without an atlas, but for most researchers these atlases are essential. Moreover, the process of examining the anatomy closely leads to a better appreciation of anatomical variability, increases one's ability to correctly identify these structures in the future without reference to an atlas, and helps build up a 3D internal mental model of neuroanatomy, which we think is an essential aspect of neuroimaging expertise.

10.2.3 Probabilistic atlases

Whereas the atlases described previously are based on the brains of single individuals, a probabilistic atlas attempts to provide a description of the variability in the localization of specific anatomical structures within a stereotactic space across a large number of individuals. For example, the LONI probabilistic atlas (Shattuck et al., 2008) was created by manually labeling 56 structures in each hemisphere for a group of 40 individuals and then normalizing those data into MNI space. The data were then used to create maps that show the probability of any specific anatomical region at a particular region. A similar probabilistic atlas, based on a different manual labeling scheme and known as the Harvard-Oxford atlas, is included with FSL; the FSLView viewer also includes a set of atlas tools, which can provide for any voxel whose regions are potentially present at that voxel and their likelihood (see Figure 10.5). Because they are reflective of the variability that exists between individuals, these atlases can provide a much more reliable way to label activation locations.

10.2.4 Automated anatomical labeling

Another option for anatomical localization is the use of software capable of automatically labeling individual T1-weighted images using standard anatomical parcellation schemes (e.g., Desikan et al., 2006; Fischl et al., 2002). These techniques rely on automated methods for identifying sulci and matching them to labeled models in order to parcellate and identify anatomical regions. For example, the FreeSurfer software package can parcellate a T1-weighted high-resolution anatomical image, providing a label image identifying the anatomical region for each voxel. Similarly, the FIRST tool in FSL can produce parcellated images of subcortical structures. These tools can be very helpful when identifying anatomical regions, as well as for creating independent anatomical regions of interest. However, the labelings are not 100% accurate across individuals, and it is important to manually verify the labeling, again with reference to an atlas. This is particularly the case for regions such as the amygdala that can be very difficult to segment.

10.3 Localizing and reporting activation

Nearly all neuroimaging papers report tables with stereotactic coordinates and associated anatomical labels; an example is shown in Table 10.1. In general, these coordinates are reported in either the space defined by the Talairach atlas (which is generally referred to as Talairach space) or that defined by the MNI template

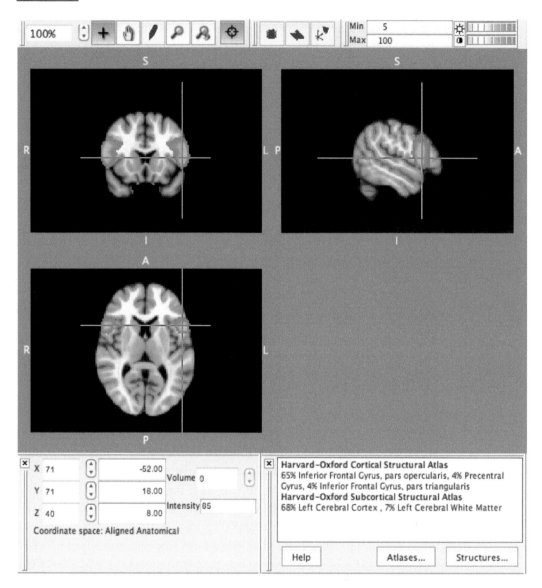

Figure 10.5. An example from the Harvard-Oxford probabilistic anatomical atlas, which is included with the FSL software package. The color map represents the likelihood of each voxel containing the structure of interest (in this case, the pars opercularis of the inferior frontal gyrus). The atlas browser (bottom right) also provides anatomical likelihood information for the selected voxel.

(which is generally referred to as MNI space). There is currently some confusion regarding what is meant by a standard space in neuroimaging publications (cf. Brett et al., 2002), which is exacerbated by the tendency to use the term "Talairach space" as a generic label for any stereotactic space, and even to use "Talairaching" as a generic verb to describe spatial normalization.

Table 10.1. An example of the tables of stereotactic coordinates usually presented in fMRI papers

Region	X (mm)	Y (mm)	Z (mm)	Maximum Z	Cluster Extent
L occipital	−12	−94	−6	3.5	124
R inf frontal	56	14	14	4.1	93
B ant cingulate	−2	32	26	3.8	110

In the early days of neuroimaging, Talairach space was the standard, but it has largely been supplanted by MNI space (for good reasons, as described earlier). Almost all major analysis packages use templates based on the MNI152 space as a default for normalization, which makes it the natural space for reporting results. For these reasons, MNI space was chosen by the International Consortium for Brain Mapping (ICBM) as the "standard" for neuroimaging experiments. However, the presence of multiple standards in the literature continues to lead to confusion, and the lack of a standard "bridge" that provides a 1:1 mapping between spaces means that noise will be introduced by any traversal across spaces. In our opinion, it makes little sense to normalize to MNI space and then convert the results to the Talairach space for reporting purposes, particularly given the aforementioned problems with the Talairach system. By adopting a single standard, the community would improve both accuracy and transparency when reporting activations.

With regard to reporting of results, it is also critical that the details of the spatial normalization procedure are described in any neuroimaging publication (cf., Poldrack et al., 2007). This should include a description of the software that is used for normalization and the parameters used with that software, such as whether the normalization was linear or nonlinear and how many parameters were used in the transformation. In addition, the specific target used for normalization should be specified (e.g., "the data were spatially normalized to the MNI avg152 T1-weighted template using a 12-parameter affine transformation with FLIRT"). These details are particularly important given that there appear to be differences in the resulting stereotactic spaces between different versions of the MNI template and different normalization software (Van Essen & Dierker, 2007). AFNI users should note that if the automatic Talairach registration (auto_tlrc) procedure is used, the coordinates are not true Talairach coordinates, since they are generated from an MNI template that has been modified to match the Talairach atlas using an unspecified transformation. Thus, it is critical that AFNI users specifically report which registration procedure was used.

10.3.1 Reporting Brodmann's areas

In neuroimaging papers, activations are often reported in terms of Brodmann's areas (BA) in addition to macroanatomical structure. One commonly used approach is to determine BA labels based on the Talairach atlas, either manually or using automated means such as the Talairach Daemon. However, as previously discussed, the BA labels in the Talairach atlas are actually just "guesstimates" about the actual location of Brodmann's areas. Another approach is to infer BA labels from macroanatomy using Brodmann's original map as a guide; for example, activation in the triangular portion of the inferior frontal gyrus is often assigned to BA45 based on their correspondence in Brodmann's original atlas. However, it is now clear that cytoarchitecture does not map cleanly onto macroanatomy; in particular, borders of Brodmann's areas do not match sulcal boundaries, and there is substantial variability in the relation between Brodmann's areas and macroanatomy (Amunts et al., 1999). Consequently, informal estimates of Brodmann areas are unwarranted and should be avoided (Uylings et al., 2005).

A more valid method is to use the probabilistic BA maps generated by Zilles and colleagues. These maps (available in standard image formats normalized to the MNI space) are based on post-mortem histology from multiple brains, yielding a probabilistic estimate of locations that explicitly includes variability. These atlases are now available within both SPM (via the SPM Anatomy Toolbox; Eickhoff et al., 2005) and FSL (as part of the FSLView atlas toolkit), which allows the integration of these maps with functional imaging analysis. The limitation of this approach is that, due to the painstakingly difficult nature of this work, these maps only exist for a small subset of BAs, so it may not be possible to identify all of the BAs for a set of activations in a study.

Finally, it should be noted that the use of Brodmann's areas is based on the assumption that they reflect functionally important boundaries. However, this assumption may not be correct. As noted by Orban & Vanduffel (2007), it is well known that individual Brodmann's areas (e.g., area 18 in the visual cortex) exhibit substantial functional heterogeneity, suggesting that even if cytoarchitecture were known for human subjects (which is it not), it may not be the best guide to function.

10.3.2 Creating coordinate lists

It is customary to report multiple local maxima for larger clusters; for example, users of SPM generally report the top three local maxima since that is the number of maxima reported by default in the software's output. It is important to note that when clusters are very large, this limitation to a small number of maxima can lead to a description that leaves out many structures that may be activated. However, reporting every possible maximum within the cluster can result in unwieldy tables of coordinates. Another alternative is to provide for each cluster a listing of all of the anatomical regions that are encompassed by the cluster. For example, one could intersect the cluster with a probabilistic atlas image and report all of the regions that fall within the cluster. This results in a more faithful anatomical description, but has the drawback that any regions not included in the table will not be included in coordinate-based meta-analyses that may be performed based on the data.

10.4 Region of interest analysis

In a region of interest analysis, the fMRI signal is characterized within a defined region and analyzed as an aggregate rather than voxel by voxel. One might want to perform an ROI analysis for several reasons, which have very different justifications and make very different assumptions. One reason is to control for Type I error by limiting the number of statistical tests to a few ROIs. A second reason is to limit testing to a region that is functionally defined on the basis of some other information, such as a separate "localizer" scan or condition. Finally, ROI analysis can be used to characterize the patterns that led to a significant result. In complex designs, such as factorial designs with multiple levels, it can often be difficult to discern the pattern of activity across conditions from an overall statistical map, and it can be useful to see the signal in areas of interest plotted for each condition.

10.4.1 ROIs for statistical control

Because whole-brain correction of familywise error can be quite conservative, it is often preferable to limit the analysis to predefined ROIs, thus reducing the number of statistical tests to be controlled for. In SPM parlance, this is known as *small volume correction*. This approach is only to be used in cases where the region of interest was specified before *any* analysis has been performed on the data. If any knowledge of the results leaks into the choice of small volumes, then the resulting statistical results will be biased, inflating familywise Type I error. We recommend that prior to analyzing any dataset, one writes down a set of anatomical ROIs that are hypothesized to be involved for each contrast. Although it is perfectly acceptable to base small volume corrections on the results from previous studies, it is *not acceptable* to look to previous studies and choose regions after a dataset has been analyzed, since the choice of regions from the prior studies will be biased by the known results.

10.4.2 Defining ROIs

ROIs can be defined either in terms of structural or functional features. Structural ROIs are generally defined based on macroanatomy, such as gyral anatomy. In many cases, the best practice is to define such ROIs for each subject based on their own anatomy, since there can be substantial variability between individuals in macroscopic anatomy. Recent developments in automated anatomical labeling offer the promise of highly reliable labeling of cortical and subcortical structures in individual anatomical images with a minimum of manual intervention (Fischl et al., 2002), though it will remain important to confirm these results against the actual anatomy. One common practice that requires extreme caution is the use of ROIs based on single-subject anatomical atlases, such as the AAL atlas (Tzourio-Mazoyer et al., 2002) or the Talairach atlas. Because of the inability of spatial normalization to perfectly match brains across individuals, there will be substantial lack of overlap

> **Box 10.4.2** Circularity and "voodoo correlations"
>
> In 2009, a paper ignited a firestorm in the fMRI community over ROI analysis methods. Originally titled "Voodoo Correlations in Social Neuroscience," the paper by Vul et al. (2009) accused a large number of studies of engaging in circular data analysis practices that led to greatly inflated estimates of effect sizes. The paper focused on findings of correlations between behavioral measures (such as personality tests) and activation, but the point holds for any study that attempts to estimate the size of an activation effect using a region of interest derived from the same data. Around the same time, Kriegeskorte et al. (2009) published a paper that more generally outlined the problem of "circular analysis" in neuroscience (not limited to neuroimaging).
>
> The circular analysis problem arises when one selects a subset of noisy variables (e.g., voxels) from an initial analysis for further characterization. When a voxel exceeds the threshold (and is thus selected for further analysis), this can be due either to signal or to noise. In the case in which there is no signal, the only voxels that will exceed the threshold will be the ones that have a very strong positive noise value. If we then estimate the mean intensity of only those voxels that exceed the threshold, they will necessarily have a large positive value; there is no way that it could be otherwise, since they were already selected on the basis of exceeding the threshold. In the case where there is both true signal and noise, the mean of the voxels that exceed threshold will be inflated by the positive noise values, since those voxels with strong negative noise contributions will not reach threshold. Thus, the mean effect size for voxels reaching threshold will over-estimate the true effect size.
>
> The review by Vul et al. (2009) suggested that a large number of studies in the social neuroscience literature had used circular analysis methods to determine effect sizes, and that these estimates were thus inflated. Although the published responses to that paper raised various issues, none disputed the prevalence or problematic nature of circular analysis in the fMRI literature. Since the publication of these papers, the literature has become much more sensitive to the issue of circularity, and it is now generally unacceptable.

between any group of subjects and these atlases (Nieto-Castanon et al., 2003). If it is necessary to use atlas-based ROIs (i.e., anatomical ROIs not derived from one's own subjects), then the best practice is to use ROIs based on probabilistic atlases of macroscopic anatomy (Hammers et al., 2003; Shattuck et al., 2008) or probabilistic cytoarchitectural atlases (Eickhoff et al., 2005).

Functional ROIs are generally based on analysis of data from the same individual. The "gold standard" approach is to use an independent functional *localizer* scan to identify voxels in a particular anatomical region that show a particular response. For example, in studies of visual processing, it is common to perform separate scans to first identify retinotopically responsive regions of visual cortex, and then analyze the data from other scans separately using retinotopically defined areas as ROIs. This is an optimal approach because the localizer is completely independent of the data being analyzed. It has been argued that functional ROIs can alternatively be created using an orthogonal contrast in the same design (Friston et al., 2006). However, it has been shown by Kriegeskorte et al. (2009) that this procedure can result in bias in the resulting estimates if the "effective regressors" defined by the contrasts are not orthogonal (which can occur due to correlations between conditions in rapid event-related designs).

One additional way that ROIs can be created is based on previous studies. Although one can take the stereotactic coordinates from an activation in a single study and place an ROI at that location, it is better practice to derive ROIs from meta-analyses of the domain or task of interest. There are now well-established methods for meta-analysis of functional imaging studies (e.g., Costafreda, 2009), and these methods can be used to generate ROIs that will be more reliable than those based on single-study activations.

10.4.3 Quantifying signals within an ROI

Once an ROI has been defined, it is then necessary to quantify the fMRI signal within the region. There are a number of approaches to this problem.

10.4.3.1 Voxel-counting

One approach that was often used in early studies is to threshold the statistical map and count the number of activated voxels in each region. However, this approach is problematic, as it can be very sensitive to the specific threshold. Further, voxel counts have been shown to be an unreliable measure of activation compared to direct measures of signal change (Cohen & DuBois, 1999). A more common approach is to use some form of summary statistic across voxels in the region of interest.

10.4.3.2 Extracting signals for ROI analysis

Data are commonly extracted for ROI analysis in two ways. In *parameter estimate extraction*, one extracts the estimated parameter value (e.g., "beta" images in SPM, "pe" images in FSL) for each condition in the statistical model. This can be particularly useful for understanding contrasts that include a number of conditions (e.g., multiway interactions in ANOVA models), but it does not provide any new information beyond that contained in the standard analysis beyond collapsing across voxels within the region.

In *hemodynamic response extraction*, the raw data are interrogated and the entire hemodynamic response to each condition across the ROI is estimated, generally using a finite impulse response (FIR) model that estimates the evoked response at each point in peristimulus time (Dale, 1999); see Section 5.1.2.2 for more on this model. This approach provides a different view of the data by showing the entire estimated response in time (making no assumptions about its shape), rather than the fit of an assumed hemodynamic response. The FIR model can tend to overfit the data given the large number of parameters (one for each timepoint in the hemodynamic response), and thus one can sometimes see estimated hemodynamic responses that are not physiologically plausible, especially with smaller sample sizes. Approaches using constrained flexible basis sets such as smoothed FIR (Goutte et al., 2000), logistic models (Lindquist & Wager, 2007), or optimized basis sets (Woolrich et al., 2004a) may be useful for obtaining better estimates of the underlying hemodynamic response.

It is not uncommon for papers to present figures showing hemodynamic responses estimated from regions that were active in a statistical model that was based on an assumed hemodynamic response; the implication is that the shape of the resulting data provides some confidence that the data conform to the expected shape of a hemodynamic response. However, such analyses are circular; because the analysis searched for regions that showed responses that resemble a canonical HRF, it would be impossible for the response in significant regions not to show a response that resembles the canonical HRF.

10.4.3.3 Computing percent signal change

Rather than using raw parameter estimate values, it is usually preferable to compute a more standard measure, and the most common is the percentage of BOLD signal change. This measure is simply the magnitude of the BOLD response divided by the overall mean of the BOLD time series. For a single trial type, the magnitude of the BOLD signal is the change in BOLD from baseline to peak of the response. The parameter estimates obtained from the GLM are not direct measures of the magnitude of the BOLD response, but a scaled version dependent on the height of the regressor used in the model. Consider a study using blocked trials, where each block has the same number of trials. The estimated signal from the GLM parameter estimates would be given by $\hat{\beta}_0 + X\hat{\beta}_1$, where $\hat{\beta}_0$ is the estimated intercept, X is the regressor for the blocked task, and $\hat{\beta}_1$ is the corresponding parameter estimate. Therefore, the estimated magnitude of the BOLD signal would be given by the height of the regressor, X, multiplied by the parameter estimate, $\hat{\beta}_1$. So, the value for percent signal change would be given by $PCH = 100 * PE * BM/MN$, where PE is the GLM parameter estimate, BM is the distance from the baseline to maximum of the regressor, and MN is the mean of the BOLD time series and multiplication by 100 puts the value into percentage units. Note that this is a very simple case where the stimuli are blocked in blocks of equal length.

Two issues arise when stimuli are of varying lengths or when the ISI varies between trials. First, due to the linearity of the relationship between the neural response and BOLD signal, which was discussed in Chapter 5, we know that shorter stimuli have a smaller BOLD signal than longer stimuli and this needs to be accounted for in the percent signal change calculation to avoid misrepresentation of the signal strength. Second, in these types of designs, it is not clear what should be used as the regressor height in the percent signal change calculation. An incorrect approach is to use the maximum height of the regressor, which does not result in an interpretable percent signal change value. For example, let's say two investigators are using exactly the same task, but one is presenting the stimuli in a slow fixed ISI design, while the other uses a random ISI presentation. Their stimulus presentation timings, GLM regressors (blue) and measured BOLD responses (red) are shown in Figure 10.6. Notice that in both cases at 20 s the studies have isolated stimuli so not only are the regressors identical in a window around this trial, but the BOLD magnitudes (and hence the GLM parameter estimates) are identical, indicating that although two different types of stimulus presentation styles were used, the BOLD activation for both studies is the same and so the estimated percent signal change values should match. If the baseline/max range of the GLM regressors were used in the percent signal change estimation, study A would yield a percent signal change of $100 * 1 * 3.85/100 = 3.85$, since the min/max range of the regressor is 1, the parameter estimate is 3.85 and the mean of the time series is 100. Study B would yield a percent signal change of $100 * 1.97 * 3.85/100 = 7.58$, since the min/max range of this regressor is 1.97. These results are clearly not identical, and therefore this approach to calculating percent signal change is not an effective or meaningful way of communicating the magnitude of a BOLD response.

To create interpretable percent signal change values, one should use the baseline to max distance of a specified event type in the calculation and report the specific event type and canonical HRF used when reporting percent signal change. Reporting the event type is analogous to measuring a distance and reporting it in inches or centimeters, since if you were to simply say the length of something was 10 there is no way to interpret this without knowing the metric used. This height should be calculated using the upsampled regressor in a higher time resolution to ensure the maximum is properly captured. If the time resolution of the TR is used, the maximum will not be properly estimated unless it falls exactly on the TR. The trial type need not occur in the actual study, as it is simply a ruler or metric used to express percent signal change. So, for example, one could use the height of the regressor that would result from convolving a 1-s long stimulus with a double gamma HRF, which is 0.2087 using the default double gamma HRF from SPM or FSL (time resolution of 0.1 s was used for the calculation). Then, in both studies shown in Figure 10.6, the percent signal change would be identical (0.18). Note that typically the baseline/max height is preferred to the min/max range in order to avoid the poststimulus undershoot. So, in general, percent signal change is given by $PCH = 100 * PE * BM/MN$, where PE is the value of the parameter estimate from the GLM, BM is the baseline max height of the trial type that is being used as a ruler for the calculation, and MN is the mean of the BOLD time series.

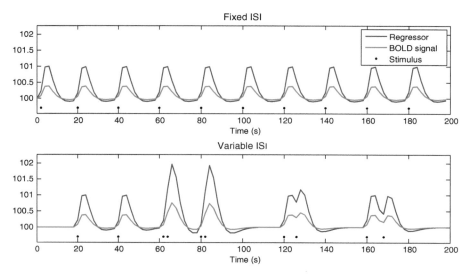

Figure 10.6. Examples of regressors and BOLD signal for two studies using the same stimuli but different stimulus presentation strategies. The study in the top image uses isolated trials and the baseline/max range of the regressor is 1. The second study uses a variable ISI and so the baseline/max range of the regressor is larger (1.97) due to two trials that are close in time. Although the brain activity has the same magnitude in both studies, as can be seen at 20 s, where both studies have an isolated 2-s trial, using the baseline/max range to calculate percent signal change will incorrectly give different results.

The preceding example deals with the calculation of percent signal change for a single task, but typically fMRI studies focus on contrasts of parameter estimates for different tasks. Say, for example, the first two regressors in the GLM modeled faces and houses, respectively, and we estimated the contrast $c = [1 \ -1]$ to find activation related to faces minus houses. Now we would like to report the activation in terms of percent signal change. It might be tempting to simply use the equation $PCH = 100 * CON * BM/MN$, replacing the parameter estimate of the previous equation with the contrast estimate $CON = c\hat{\beta}$, but this could produce misleading estimates. Consider the case where one investigator used the contrast $c_1 = [1 \ -1]$ and another used $c_2 = [2 \ -2]$. Although both of these contrasts are valid and will result in identical inferences, the first contrast estimate, $c_1\hat{\beta}$, will be half as large as the second contrast estimate, $c_2\hat{\beta}$. Since the interpretation of the second contrast is twice the difference of faces and houses, the appropriate percent signal change corresponding to the difference of faces and houses would be given by $\frac{1}{2} * c_2\hat{\beta} * BM/MN$, so a contrast scale factor is introduced to ensure the interpretation of the percent signal change calculation. Specifically, $PCH = 100 * SF * CON * BM/MN$, where SF is the appropriate contrast scale factor.

Another example would be if three trial types were used and the contrast $c = [1 \ 1 \ 1]$ was used to test the activation for the average response across all three trial types. Again, this contrast is valid in terms of the hypothesis test for the mean across tasks, but the interpretation of $CON = c\hat{\boldsymbol{\beta}}$ is actually the sum of the three tasks, and so the appropriate percent signal change calculation would be given by $PCH = 100 * \frac{1}{3} CON * BM/MN$. Note that, in most cases, if contrasts are constructed so that the positive numbers in the contrast sum to 1 and the negative numbers sum to -1, the scale factor in this calculation will be 1. Exceptions include some contrasts that may arise in more complicated ANOVA models.

10.4.3.4 Summarizing data within an ROI

Once the signals have been extracted, they need to be summarized, and even this seemingly uncontroversial operation requires some careful thought. The simplest method is to simply average the extracted signal across voxels within the ROI, and this is a common method. However, within SPM, the default method is to compute the first principal component (or *eigenvariate*) of the signal. The intuition behind this method is that if there are multiple processes occurring within the region, the first principal component will reflect the strongest of those processes, whereas the mean will reflect a combination of them. The most obvious example is the case where there are both activated and deactivated voxels within a single ROI, in which case the major eigenvariate may be more reflective of the largest of those whereas the mean may be close to zero. There have not been any systematic comparisons of these methods to our knowledge, but we would note that in most cases the mean and first principal component of signals from within an ROI will be highly correlated with one another.

When large anatomical ROIs are used (e.g., the entire superior temporal gyrus), even if the region contains significantly active voxels, this activation may only occur in a small proportion of voxels in the ROI. This suggests that simply averaging across the entire region could swamp the signal from this small number of voxels with noise from the remaining nonactivated voxels. There is no widely accepted solution to this problem, which suggests that ROI analyses should focus on relatively small and/or functionally coherent regions if possible.

Appendix A: Review of the General Linear Model

The general linear model is an important tool in many fMRI data analyses. As the name "general" suggests, this model can be used for many different types of analyses, including correlations, one-sample t-tests, two-sample t-tests, analysis of variance (ANOVA), and analysis of covariance (ANCOVA). This appendix is a review of the GLM and covers parameter estimation, hypothesis testing, and model setup for these various types of analyses.

Some knowledge of matrix algebra is assumed in this section, and for a more detailed explanation of the GLM, it is recommended to read Neter et al. (1996).

A.1 Estimating GLM parameters

The GLM relates a single continuous dependent, or response, variable to one or more continuous or categorical independent variables, or predictors. The simplest model is a *simple linear regression*, which contains a single independent variable. For example, finding the relationship between the dependent variable of mental processing speed and the independent variable, age (Figure A.1). The goal is to create a model that fits the data well and since this appears to be a simple linear relationship between age and processing speed, the model is $Y = \beta_0 + \beta_1 X_1$, where Y is a vector of length T containing the processing speeds for T subjects, β_0 describes where the line crosses the y axis, β_1 is the slope of the line and X_1 is the vector of length T containing the ages of the subjects. Note that if β_0 is omitted from the model, the fitted line will be forced to go through the origin, which typically does not follow the trend of the data very well and so intercepts are included in almost all linear models.

Notice that the data points in Figure A.1 do not lie exactly in a line. This is because Y, the processing speeds, are random quantities that have been measured with some degree of error. To account for this, a random error term is added to the GLM model

$$Y = \beta_0 + \beta_1 X_1 + \epsilon$$

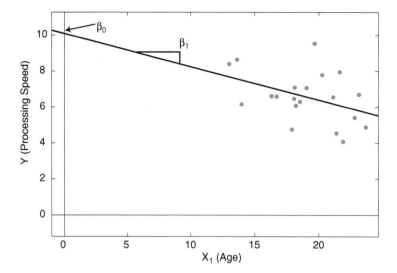

Figure A.1. Example of data and model for a simple linear regression. The intercept, β_0, is where the line crosses the y axis and the slope, β_1, describes the relationship between the dependent variable, mental processing speed, and the independent variable, age.

where ϵ is a random vector of length T that describes the distribution of the error between the true value of the dependent variable and the measured values that are obtained for the study. The standard assumption is that ϵ is normally distributed such that the vector has a mean of 0 and a variance of σ^2. Further, any two elements of the error vector are assumed to be uncorrelated, $\text{Cor}(\epsilon_i, \epsilon_j) = 0$. This is typically written as $\epsilon \sim N(0, \sigma^2 I)$, where N is the multivariate normal distribution and I is a $T \times T$ identity matrix, which only has 1s along the diagonal and 0s on the off diagonal.

The interpretation of the model follows: If we were to know the true values of β_0 and β_1, then for a given age, say 20 years old, the expected mean processing speed for this age would be $\beta_0 + \beta_1 \times 20$. If we were to collect a sample of processing speeds from 20 year olds, the distribution of the data would be normal with a mean of $\beta_0 + \beta_1 \times 20$ and a variance of σ^2. Although the mean processing speed would change for different age groups, the variance would be the same. The distribution for those with an age of 10 years would have a mean of $\beta_0 + \beta_1 \times 20$ and a variance of σ^2.

A.1.1 Simple linear regression

To find the estimates of the parameters β_0 and β_1, the method of *least squares* is used, which minimizes the squared difference between the data, Y, and the estimates, $\hat{Y} = \hat{\beta}_0 + \hat{\beta}_1 X_1$. This difference is known as the residual, and this is denoted by $e = Y - \hat{Y}$ and would be the horizontal distance between a point and the fitted line. The estimate of the error variance, σ^2, is given by $\hat{\sigma}^2 = \frac{e'e}{T-2}$, where T is the number of data points. The quantity $T - 2$ is the degrees of freedom for this model and consists of the amount of information going into the model (T data points) minus the number of parameters we had to estimate (two, β_0 and β_1). The line shown in Figure A.1 illustrates the least squares fit of the model to the data where, for a given age, the distribution of processing speed for that age is estimated to have a mean of $\hat{\beta}_0 + age \times \hat{\beta}_1$, and $\hat{\sigma}^2$ is the estimate of the variance of the data for that value of age.

Under the assumptions that the error has a mean of zero, constant variance and correlation of 0, the least squares estimates of the $\hat{\beta}_i$s have a nice property according to the Gauss Markov theorem (Graybill, 1961), which is that $\hat{\beta}$ is unbiased and has the smallest variance among all unbiased estimators of β. In other words if we were to repeat the experiment an infinite number of times and estimate $\hat{\beta}$ each time, the average of these $\hat{\beta}$s would be equal to the true value of β. Not only that, but the variance of the estimates of $\hat{\beta}$ is smaller than any other estimator that gives an unbiased estimate of β. When the assumptions are violated, the estimate will not have these properties, and Section A.3 will describe the methods used to handle these situations.

A.1.2 Multiple linear regression

It is possible to have multiple independent variables, $X_1, X_2, \ldots, X_p$, in which case the GLM would be $Y = \beta_0 + \beta_1 X_1 + \beta_2 X_2 + \cdots + \beta_p X_p + \epsilon$. The error term, ϵ, is distributed the same as before ($\epsilon \sim N(0, \sigma^2 I)$) and each parameter, β_i, is interpreted as the effect of X_i controlling for all other variables in the model. So, for example, if age and gender were independent variables, the parameter estimate for age would be the relationship of age on processing speed, adjusting for gender or holding gender constant. Sometimes the parameters in a multiple linear regression are referred to as *partial regression coefficients* since they reflect the effect of one predictor controlling for all of the other predictors.

The multiple linear regression formula can be concisely expressed using matrix algebra as

$$Y = X\boldsymbol{\beta} + \epsilon$$

where X is a $T \times p$ matrix with each column corresponding to an X_i and $\boldsymbol{\beta}$ is a column vector of length $p + 1$, $\boldsymbol{\beta} = [\beta_0, \beta_1, \cdots, \beta_p]'$. The use of matrix algebra makes the derivation of $\hat{\boldsymbol{\beta}}$ easy. Since X isn't a square matrix, we can't solve the equation $Y = X\boldsymbol{\beta}$ by premultiplying both sides by X^{-1}, because only square matrices have inverses. Instead, if we first premultiply both sides of the equation by X', we have the so-called *normal equations*

$$X'Y = X'X\boldsymbol{\beta}$$

Table A.1. Two examples of rank deficient matrices

$$
\begin{pmatrix}
1 & 0 & 7 \\
1 & 0 & 7 \\
0 & 1 & 0 \\
0 & 1 & 0
\end{pmatrix}
\qquad
\begin{pmatrix}
1 & 0 & 2 \\
1 & 0 & 2 \\
1 & 1 & 5 \\
1 & 1 & 5
\end{pmatrix}
$$

It can be shown that any $\boldsymbol{\beta}$ that satisfies the normal equations minimizes the sum-of-squares of the residuals $\mathbf{e}'\mathbf{e}$, and thus it gives the least squares solution

$$\hat{\boldsymbol{\beta}} = (\mathbf{X}'\mathbf{X})^{-1}\mathbf{X}'\mathbf{Y} \tag{A.1}$$

assuming $\mathbf{X}'\mathbf{X}$ is invertible.

The estimate for σ^2 is the same as before, $\hat{\sigma}^2 = \frac{\mathbf{e}'\mathbf{e}}{T-(p+1)}$, where T is the number of rows in X and $p+1$ is the number of columns, resulting in $T-(p+1)$ the degrees of freedom for multiple linear regression.

In order for the inverse of $\mathbf{X}'\mathbf{X}$ to exist, X must have full column rank, which means no column is a linear combination of any of the other columns in the design matrix. In Table A.1, the matrix on the left-hand side is rank deficient since multiplying the first column by 7 yields the third column, and the matrix on the right is rank deficient since twice the first column plus three times the second equals the third column. If the design matrix is rank deficient there is not a unique solution for the parameter estimates. Consider the matrix on the left of Table A.1, and estimate the three corresponding parameters, β_1, β_2, β_3, when $\mathbf{Y} = [14\ 14\ 0\ 0]'$. It is easy to show that not only are $\beta_1 = 0, \beta_2 = 0$, and $\beta_3 = 2$ parameters that give an exact solution since

$$
\begin{pmatrix}
1 & 0 & 7 \\
1 & 0 & 7 \\
0 & 1 & 0 \\
0 & 1 & 0
\end{pmatrix}
\begin{pmatrix}
0 \\
0 \\
2
\end{pmatrix}
=
\begin{pmatrix}
14 \\
14 \\
0 \\
0
\end{pmatrix}
\tag{A.2}
$$

but $\beta_1 = 14, \beta_2 = 0$, and $\beta_3 = 0$ and an infinite number of other combinations will also perfectly fit the data.

A.2 Hypothesis testing

The previous section described how to obtain the estimates of the parameters $\beta_0, \beta_1, \ldots, \beta_p$ and σ^2, and this section describes how to carry out hypothesis tests on linear combinations, or contrasts, of the β_is. A row-vector of length $p+1$ is used to define the contrast to be tested. The simplest contrast tests a single parameter in the vector of parameters, $\boldsymbol{\beta}$. For example, if there were four parameters in the model, $[\beta_0, \beta_1, \beta_2, \beta_3]'$, then the contrast to test whether the first parameter, β_0 was different from 0, $H_0 : \beta_0 = 0$, would be $\mathbf{c} = [1\ 0\ 0\ 0]$, since $\mathbf{c}\boldsymbol{\beta} = \beta_0$. It is also possible to test whether two parameters are different from each other. To test, $H_0 : \beta_2 = \beta_3$, which is equivalent to $H_0 : \beta_2 - \beta_3 = 0$, the contrast $\mathbf{c} = [0 \ 1 \ -1 \ 0]$ would be used. In both of these cases, the null hypothesis can be re-expressed as $H_0 : \mathbf{c}\boldsymbol{\beta} = 0$.

To test the hypothesis, the distribution of $\mathbf{c}\hat{\boldsymbol{\beta}}$ under the null assumption, that the contrast is equal to 0, must be known. It can be shown that the distribution of $\mathbf{c}\hat{\boldsymbol{\beta}}$ is normal with a mean of $\mathbf{c}\boldsymbol{\beta}$ and a variance of $\mathbf{c}(\mathbf{X}'\mathbf{X})^{-1}\mathbf{c}'\sigma^2$, so under the null hypothesis, $\mathbf{c}\hat{\boldsymbol{\beta}} \sim N(0, \mathbf{c}(\mathbf{X}'\mathbf{X})^{-1}\mathbf{c}'\sigma^2)$. Since we do not know the variance σ^2, we cannot use the normal distribution to carry out the hypothesis test. Instead, we use the t statistic

$$t = \frac{\mathbf{c}\hat{\boldsymbol{\beta}}}{\sqrt{\mathbf{c}(\mathbf{X}'\mathbf{X})^{-1}\mathbf{c}'\hat{\sigma}^2}} \tag{A.3}$$

which, under the null, is distributed as a t-distribution with $T - (p + 1)$ degrees of freedom. A P-value for a one-sided alternative hypothesis, such as $H_A : \mathbf{c}\boldsymbol{\beta} > 0$ is given by $P(T_{T-(p+1)} \geq t)$, where $T_{N-(p+1)}$ is a random variable following a t-distribution with $T - (p + 1)$ degrees of freedom, and t is the observed test statistic. The P-value for a two-sided hypothesis test, $H_A : \mathbf{c}\boldsymbol{\beta} \neq 0$, is calculated as $P(T_{T-(p+1)} \geq |t|)$.

In addition to hypothesis testing of single contrasts using a t-statistic, one can also simultaneously test multiple contrasts using an F-test. For example, again using the model with four parameters, to test whether all of the βs are 0, $H_0 : \beta_1 = \beta_2 = \beta_3 = \beta_4 = 0$, one would specify a set of contrasts in the form of a matrix. Each row of the contrast corresponds to one of the four simultaneous tests, in this case that a particular β_i is 0, and looks like the following:

$$\mathbf{c} = \begin{pmatrix} 1 & 0 & 0 & 0 \\ 0 & 1 & 0 & 0 \\ 0 & 0 & 1 & 0 \\ 0 & 0 & 0 & 1 \end{pmatrix} \tag{A.4}$$

The F-statistic is then given by

$$F = (\mathbf{c}\hat{\boldsymbol{\beta}})'[r\mathbf{c}\left(\widehat{\mathrm{Cov}}(\hat{\boldsymbol{\beta}})\right)\mathbf{c}']^{-1}(\mathbf{c}\hat{\boldsymbol{\beta}}) \tag{A.5}$$

where r is the rank of $\mathbf{c}$ and typically is equal to the number of rows in $\mathbf{c}$. The F-statistic in Equation (A.5) is distributed as an F with r numerator and $T - (p+1)$ denominator degrees of freedom $(F_{r,T-(p+1)})$.

A.3 Correlation and heterogeneous variances

One of the important assumptions of the GLM, mentioned at the beginning of this appendix, is that the elements of the error vector, ϵ are uncorrelated, $\mathrm{Cor}(\epsilon_i, \epsilon_j) = 0$ for $i \neq j$ and that they all have the same variance, $\mathrm{Var}(\epsilon_i) = \sigma^2$ for all i. There are many cases when this assumption is violated. For example, imagine that the dataset on age and processing speed included sets of identical twins; in this case, some individuals will be more similar than others. More relevant to fMRI, this can also occur when the dependent variable Y includes temporally correlated data. When this occurs, the distribution of the error is given by $\text{Cov}(\epsilon) = \sigma^2 \mathbf{V}$, where $\mathbf{V}$ is the symmetric correlation matrix and σ^2 is the varaince.

The most common solution to this problem is to *prewhiten* the data, or to remove the temporal correlation. Since a correlation matrix is symmetric and positive definite, the Cholesky decomposition can be used to find a matrix $\mathbf{K}$ such that $\mathbf{V}^{-1} = \mathbf{K}'\mathbf{K}$ (see Harville (1997) for more details on matrix decomposition). To prewhiten the data, $\mathbf{K}$ is premultiplied on both sides of the GLM to give

$$\mathbf{KY} = \mathbf{KX}\boldsymbol{\beta} + \mathbf{K}\epsilon \tag{A.6}$$

Since the errors are now independent,

$$\text{Cov}(\mathbf{K}\epsilon) = \mathbf{K}\text{Cov}(\epsilon)\mathbf{K}' = \sigma^2 \mathbf{I}$$

we can rewrite Equation (A.6) as

$$\mathbf{Y}^* = \mathbf{X}^*\boldsymbol{\beta} + \epsilon^* \tag{A.7}$$

where $\mathbf{Y}^* = \mathbf{KY}$, $\mathbf{X}^* = \mathbf{KX}$, and $\epsilon^* = \mathbf{K}\epsilon$. Most important, since $\text{Cov}(\epsilon^*) = \sigma^2 \mathbf{I}$, the previously stated assumptions hold, and we can use least squares to estimate our parameters and their variances. The parameter estimates would be

$$\hat{\boldsymbol{\beta}} = (\mathbf{X}^{*'}\mathbf{X}^*)^{-1}\mathbf{X}^{*'}\mathbf{Y}^* \tag{A.8}$$

which can be also written as $\hat{\boldsymbol{\beta}} = (\mathbf{X}'\mathbf{V}^{-1}\mathbf{X})^{-1}\mathbf{X}'\mathbf{V}^{-1}\mathbf{Y}$. The covariance of $\hat{\boldsymbol{\beta}}$ is given by

$$\widehat{\text{Cov}}(\hat{\boldsymbol{\beta}}) = (\mathbf{X}^{*'}\mathbf{X}^*)^{-1}\hat{\sigma}^2 \tag{A.9}$$

or $\widehat{\text{Cov}}(\hat{\boldsymbol{\beta}}) = (\mathbf{X}\mathbf{V}^{-1}\mathbf{X})^{-1}\hat{\sigma}^2$ and $\hat{\sigma}^2$ is estimated as shown earlier.

If the error terms are uncorrelated, $\text{Cor}(\epsilon) = \mathbf{I}$, but the assumption of equal variances is violated, $\text{Var}(\epsilon_i) \neq \text{Var}(\epsilon_j)$, $i \neq j$, the variances are said to be heterogeneous, and the GLM is estimated as shown in Equations (A.8) and (A.9), with $\mathbf{K} = \text{diag}(1/\sigma_1, 1/\sigma_2, \ldots, 1/\sigma_T)$. The expression $\text{diag}(1/\sigma_1, \ldots, 1/\sigma_T)$ simply refers to a matrix with 0s on the off diagonal and $1/\sigma_1, 1/\sigma_2, \ldots, 1/\sigma_T$ along the diagonal. This is known as weighted linear regression. In both the prewhitening approach and the weighted linear regression approach, the necessary variance and covariance parameters are estimated from the data and then used to get the contrast estimates and carry out hypothesis testing.

A.4 Why "general" linear model?

The GLM is a powerful tool, since many different types of analyses can be carried out using it including: one-sample t-tests, two-sample t-tests, paired t-tests, ANOVA, and ANCOVA. The first section illustrated simple linear regression in the example where processing speed was modeled as a function of age. Figure A.2 shows some common analyses that are carried out using the GLM where the top example is the simplest model, a one-sample t-test. In this case, we have one group and are interested in testing whether the overall mean is 0. The design is simply a column of 1s and the contrast is $c = [1]$.

The next design shown in Figure A.2 is a two-sample t-test, where the data either belong to group 1 (G1) or group 2 (G2). In the outcome vector, Y, all G1 observations are at the beginning, and G2 observations follow. The design matrix has two columns, where the parameter for each column corresponds to the means for G1 and G2, respectively. The contrast shown tests whether the means of the two groups are equal, but it is also possible to test the mean of each group using the separate contrasts, $c = [1\ 0]$ and $c = [0\ 1]$. Note that there are alternative ways of setting up the design for a two-sample t-test, which are not illustrated in the figure. Two other examples of design matrices for the two-sample t-test are given as X_{T1} and X_{T2} in Equation (A.10).

$$X_{T1} = \begin{pmatrix} 1 & 0 \\ \vdots & \vdots \\ 1 & 0 \\ 1 & 1 \\ \vdots & \vdots \\ 1 & 1 \end{pmatrix} \quad X_{T2} = \begin{pmatrix} 1 & 1 \\ \vdots & \vdots \\ 1 & 1 \\ 1 & -1 \\ \vdots & \vdots \\ 1 & -1 \end{pmatrix} \tag{A.10}$$

In X_{T1}, the first column models the mean of the *baseline* or unmodeled group mean. In this case, the mean of group 1 is not explicitly modeled and so the parameter corresponding to the first column would be the mean for group 1, and the parameter associated with the second column would be the difference in means between groups 1 and 2.

In the case of X_{T2} the first column corresponds to the overall mean of the data and the second column is the difference between the means of group 1 and group 2. It is often the case that there are multiple ways of setting up a design matrix, so it is important to understand what the parameters for the columns of the design correspond to. For X_{T1}, for example, $X_{T1}\boldsymbol{\beta}$ would yield the vector, $\hat{Y} = [\beta_0, \beta_0, \ldots, \beta_0, \beta_0 + \beta_1, \ldots, \beta_0 + \beta_1]'$, and so it is clear to see that β_0 corresponds to the mean of group 1 and $\beta_0 + \beta_1$ is the mean for group 2, hence β_1 is the difference between the two means. Similarly, $X_{T2}\boldsymbol{\beta}$ gives a value of $\beta_0 + \beta_1$ for the group 1 entries and $\beta_0 - \beta_1$ for the group 2 entries, meaning β_0 is the overall mean and β_1 is the difference in means between the two groups.

Test Description	Order of data	$X\beta$	Hypothesis Test
One-sample t-test. 6 observations	G_1 G_2 G_3 G_4 G_5 G_6	$\begin{pmatrix} 1 \\ 1 \\ 1 \\ 1 \\ 1 \\ 1 \end{pmatrix}\begin{bmatrix}\beta_1\end{bmatrix}$	H_0: Overall mean=0 H_0: $\beta_1 = 0$ H_0: $c\beta = 0$ $c = [1]$
Two-sample t-test. 5 subjects in group 1 (G1) and 5 subjects in group 2 (G2)	$G1_1$ $G1_2$ $G1_3$ $G1_4$ $G1_5$ $G2_1$ $G2_2$ $G2_3$ $G2_4$ $G2_5$	$\begin{pmatrix} 1 & 0 \\ 1 & 0 \\ 1 & 0 \\ 1 & 0 \\ 1 & 0 \\ 0 & 1 \\ 0 & 1 \\ 0 & 1 \\ 0 & 1 \\ 0 & 1 \end{pmatrix}\begin{bmatrix}\beta_{G1} \\ \beta_{G2}\end{bmatrix}$	H_0: mean of G1 different from G2 H_0: $\beta_{G1} - \beta_{G2} = 0$ H_0: $c\beta = 0$ $c = [1\ \ -1]$
Paired t-test. 5 paired measures of A and B.	A_{S1} B_{S1} A_{S2} B_{S2} A_{S3} B_{S3} A_{S4} B_{S4} A_{S5} B_{S5}	$\begin{pmatrix} 1 & 1 & 0 & 0 & 0 & 0 \\ -1 & 1 & 0 & 0 & 0 & 0 \\ 1 & 0 & 1 & 0 & 0 & 0 \\ -1 & 0 & 1 & 0 & 0 & 0 \\ 1 & 0 & 0 & 1 & 0 & 0 \\ -1 & 0 & 0 & 1 & 0 & 0 \\ 1 & 0 & 0 & 0 & 1 & 0 \\ -1 & 0 & 0 & 0 & 1 & 0 \\ 1 & 0 & 0 & 0 & 0 & 1 \\ -1 & 0 & 0 & 0 & 0 & 1 \end{pmatrix}\begin{pmatrix}\beta_{diff} \\ \beta_{S1} \\ \beta_{S2} \\ \beta_{S3} \\ \beta_{S4} \\ \beta_{S5}\end{pmatrix}$	H_0: A is different from B H_0: $\beta_{diff} = 0$ H_0: $c\beta = 0$ $c = [1\ 0\ 0\ 0\ 0\ 0]$
Two way ANOVA. Factor A has two levels and factor B has 3 levels. There are 2 observations for each A/B combination.	$A1B1_1$ $A1B1_2$ $A1B2_1$ $A1B2_2$ $A1B3_1$ $A1B3_2$ $A2B1_1$ $A2B1_2$ $A2B2_1$ $A2B2_2$ $A2B3_1$ $A2B3_2$	$\begin{pmatrix} 1 & 1 & 1 & 0 & 1 & 0 \\ 1 & 1 & 1 & 0 & 1 & 0 \\ 1 & 1 & 0 & 1 & 0 & 1 \\ 1 & 1 & 0 & 1 & 0 & 1 \\ 1 & 1 & -1 & -1 & -1 & -1 \\ 1 & 1 & -1 & -1 & -1 & -1 \\ 1 & -1 & 1 & 0 & -1 & 0 \\ 1 & -1 & 1 & 0 & -1 & 0 \\ 1 & -1 & 0 & 1 & 0 & -1 \\ 1 & -1 & 0 & 1 & 0 & -1 \\ 1 & -1 & -1 & -1 & 1 & 1 \\ 1 & -1 & -1 & -1 & 1 & 1 \end{pmatrix}\begin{pmatrix}\beta_{mean} \\ \beta_{A1} \\ \beta_{B1} \\ \beta_{B2} \\ \beta_{A1B1} \\ \beta_{A1B2}\end{pmatrix}$	F-tests for all contrasts H_0: Overall mean=0 H_0: $\beta_{mean} = 0$ H_0: $c\beta = 0$ $c = [1\ 0\ 0\ 0\ 0\ 0]$ H_0: Main A effect=0 H_0: $\beta_{A1} = 0$ H_0: $c\beta = 0$ $c = [0\ 1\ 0\ 0\ 0\ 0]$ H_0: Main B effect = 0 H_0: $\beta_{B1} = \beta_{B2} = 0$ H_0: $c\beta=0$ $c = \begin{bmatrix} 0 & 0 & 1 & 0 & 0 & 0 \\ 0 & 0 & 0 & 1 & 0 & 0 \end{bmatrix}$ H_0: A/B interaction effect=0 H_0: $\beta_{A1B1} = \beta_{A1B2} = 0$ H_0: $c\beta=0$ $c = \begin{bmatrix} 0 & 0 & 0 & 0 & 1 & 0 \\ 0 & 0 & 0 & 0 & 0 & 1 \end{bmatrix}$

Figure A.2. Examples of GLM models for popular study designs including: One-sample t-test, two-sample t-test, paired t-test, and two-way ANOVA. The first column describes the model, the second column describes how the data are ordered in the outcome vector, the third column shows the design matrix, and the last column illustrates the hypothesis tests and corresponding contrasts. Note, in the ANOVA example F-tests are used for all contrasts, whereas t-tests are used for the other examples.

The paired t-test is the third example in Figure A.2, where there are N groups of paired observations. For example, we could have N subjects scanned on two sessions and want to compare session 2 to session 1. In the outcome vector, Y, observations are ordered by subject, session 1 followed by session 2. The first column of the design matrix is modeling the difference and the last N columns of the design matrix are modeling subject-specific means. By adjusting for the subject-specific means, the difference refers to the difference in the *centered* or demeaned pairs of data points. To test the paired difference, the contrast only includes the first parameter, the rest of the parameters related to the subject-specific means are considered "nuisance," since we do not typically test them, but they are necessary to include in the model to pick up extra variability due to each subject having a different mean.

The last example illustrates a two-way ANOVA, with two levels for the first factor and three levels for the second factor. There are a couple of ways to set up this model, but the one illustrated here is a *factor effects* setup and is used when the interest is in testing the typical ANOVA hypotheses of overall mean, main effects, and interaction effects. In general, the format used to create the regressors is as follows: For each factor the number of regressors is equal to one less than the number of levels for that factor. So our first factor, call it A, will have one regressor associated with it and the second factor, call it B, will have two. Each regressor is modeling the difference between a level of the factor to a baseline level. For example, the second column of X in the ANOVA panel of Figure A.2 is the regressor for factor A and takes a value of 1 for rows corresponding to level 1 of A (A1), and since the second level is the reference level, all rows corresponding to A2 are -1. The third and fourth columns are the regressors for factor B and the third level, B3, is the reference so both regressors are -1 for those corresponding rows. The third regressor compares B1 to B3, so it is 1 for level B1 and 0 for level B2. The fourth regressor compares B2 to B3 and so it is 0 for B1 and 1 for B2. The last two columns make up the interaction and are found by multiplying the second and third and second and fourth columns, respectively. All contrasts are tested using an F-test, since this is standard for ANOVA. To test the main effects, we simply include a contrast for each regressor corresponding to that factor, and to test the interaction we would include a contrast for each regressor corresponding to an interaction. The other option is to use a *cell means* approach, where we simply have six regressors, one for each of the six cells of the 2×3 ANOVA. It is an extension of the two-sample t-test model shown in Figure A.2 and is more convenient when we are interested in testing hypothesis that compare the means between cells of the ANOVA.

It should be noted that in some cases it is possible to use a linear regression model when there are repeated measures. For example, the two-sample t-test can be thought of as a one-way ANOVA with two levels and repeated measures across the levels. In a similar fashion, the two-factor ANOVA model in the bottom panel of Figure A.2 can be extended to a repeated measures case, where measures are repeated for *all* factors in the model, say a subject is studied before and after a treatment (factor A) for three types of memory tasks (factor B). In this case, the single mean column would be broken up into separate subject means, and these columns of the design matrix would be treated as nuisance. A very important note when using the linear model for repeated measures ANOVA designs is that it *only* works in the case when the measures are *balanced* across the factor levels. So, for example, if a subject was missing measurements for the second and third levels of factor B after treatment, this linear regression approach cannot be used. In cases such as this, more complicated models and estimation strategies are necessary to achieve appropriate test statistics and hypothesis test results.

Appendix B: Data organization and management

The amount of computation that is performed, and data that are produced, in the process of fMRI research can be quite astounding. For a laboratory with multiple researchers, it becomes critical to ensure that a common scheme is used to organize the data; for example, when a student leaves a laboratory, the PI may still need to determine which data were used for a particular analysis reported in a paper in order to perform additional analyses. In this appendix, we discuss some practices that help researchers meet the computational needs of fMRI research and keep the data deluge under control, particularly as they move toward developing a research group or laboratory with multiple researchers performing data analysis.

B.1 Computing for fMRI analysis

The power of today's computers means that almost all of the data analysis methods discussed in this book can be performed on a standard desktop machine. Given this, one model for organization of a laboratory is what we might call "just a bunch of workstations" (JBOW). Under this model, each member of the research group has his or her own workstation on which to perform analyses. This model has the benefit of requiring little in the way of specialized hardware, system administration, or user training. Thus, one can get started very quickly with analysis. However, it has a number of potential disadvantages:

- The processing power of each individual is limited to that of a single workstation, making large analyses difficult.
- The data storage is generally not redundant, and thus failure of a single hard drive can lead to complete data loss.
- Centralized backup and archiving of the data can be difficult to organize.
- Software updates may differ across machines, such that different members of the team may use different software versions.

Another more complicated model is referred to as the client/server model, in which a centralized server provides computing resources to all of the members of the group.

This generally requires that individuals log into a central system and perform their analyses remotely. The data storage in such a system generally relies upon RAID (redundant array of inexpensive disks) storage, which provides protection against disk failure as well as faster speed by spreading files across multiple disks. The client/server model has the disadvantage of being more costly to install and difficult to administer, generally requiring professional system administration. However, it has a number of distinct advantages over the JBOW model:

- It allows one to take advantage of a large number of processors.
- The use of RAID provides better protection and lessens the impact of disk failure.
- It makes centralized backup much easier since the data reside on a single filesystem.
- It allows better control over software updating and versioning.

One recent development for fMRI analysis is the more common implementation of *grid computing*, in which a large cluster of computers can be used in parallel to perform data analysis with much greater speed than is possible with a single system. Software packages such as the Sun Grid Engine (SGE) allow parallel processing on nearly any cluster of computers, and fMRI analysis packages are beginning to provide direct support for such grid processing. For example, with FSL one can execute a large number of analysis jobs (many more than the number of processors available), and if SGE is installed, the jobs will be automatically coordinated so that the computer does not get overloaded. For these reasons, we strongly recommend that researchers adopt a client/server computing model as they start to develop a larger research group.

Operating systems.   Although there are certainly a large number of labs that effectively use Microsoft Windows for data analysis, it is our opinion that UNIX-based operating systems (e.g., Linux, Mac OS X) are the best choice for fMRI data analysis. First, there is a greater amount of freely available analysis software for UNIX systems, in comparison to Windows systems. All of the major packages (SPM, FSL, AFNI) are available for UNIX systems, whereas only SPM is can run natively on Windows. It is possible to run FSL or AFNI using a virtual machine under Windows, but this is suboptimal from a performance standpoint. Second, the ability to script analyses under UNIX is (in our opinion) superior to that under Windows systems.

B.2 Data organization

One of the most important lessons that we have learned in doing fMRI research is the need for a consistent and clear scheme for organizing and naming data files. It may seem relatively unimportant for a single study, but as datasets multiply, it becomes increasingly important to be able to find data across studies. In addition, the use of consistent data organization and naming schemes across studies allows one to relatively easily write scripts to perform analyses across multiple studies.

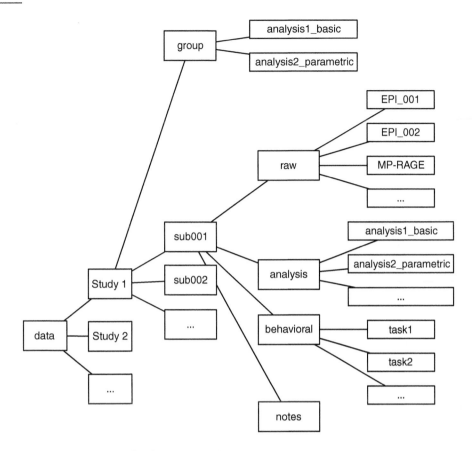

Figure B.1. Example of a schema for data organization.

One effective way to implement good data organization is to create a complete directory structure when the data are first downloaded from the MRI scanner. Figure B.1 shows an example of the data organization created by the script that is used for downloading data in one of our labs. In the process of analyzing a dataset, one often fits a number of different models to the data; we have found it very useful to place each separate model in a separate folder, with a name that is descriptive of the particular model.

Because raw fMRI data files can be quite large, it is advisable to avoid copying them multiple times for different analyses. One very useful feature of UNIX operating systems is the ability to create *symbolic links*, which are similar to file shortcuts in Windows and aliases in MacOS, and consist of a small file that points a file to another file. Symbolic links allow one to leave raw files with their original names but then create more intuitively named references to the data. It is also generally advisable to make the raw data files read-only, so that they will not be modified by any subsequent processing operations, or accidentally deleted.

For larger laboratories, there are more complicated systems available to assist with data organization. For example, the Extensible Neuroimaging Archive Toolkit (XNAT) project (http://www.xnat.org/) provides a very powerful open-source toolbox for the storage and management of neuroimaging data. Tools such as XNAT have the benefit of scaling well to very large datasets, but they also require substantial system administration expertise in order to customize them to any particular application.

B.3 Project management

As the size of one's laboratory increases, it can become increasingly difficult to determine the status of individual projects. For example, on more than one occasion we have found it necessary to track down data to create a figure for a presentation when the student who performed the analysis was not available. This can result in a challenging exercise in data archaeology. The use of consistent and transparent naming schemes for analyses can certainly help with this problem, but the challenge remains that much of the important information remains hidden in the researcher's notebook. Likewise, when a laboratory has multiple active human research protocols, it can be challenging to simply keep track of all of these.

We have found it very useful to maintain an online project management system in order to provide a permanent accessible record of all of the projects performed in the laboratory. Although there are a number of very powerful project management systems available, a simple but very useful approach is to use freely available wiki software (such as MediaWiki: http://www.mediawiki.org) to create an online repository for information about studies in the laboratory. Because editing of wiki pages is relatively simple, this provides an easy means for researchers to document their studies and analyses. It is also easy to upload files to the system. In addition, the security features of wiki software allow one to limit access to this information to the relevant lab members or guests.

It is also possible to create more direct connections between the data analysis software and the wiki system. For example, we have created software that automatically generates a wiki page whenever a subject's data are transferred from the scanner to the data analysis system. The DICOM header for each subject is transferred into a SQL database, and this information is used to create a page that shows the scan meta-data for each imaging series collected during the session. This software is freely available via the book Web site.

We suggest the following as a minimum list of information that should be included in the project management page for each project or study:

- A list of all personnel involved in the study and their individual roles in the project.
- Specific information about the location (directory and computer) of the data for each subject
- Notes regarding the exclusion of any particular subjects from the analysis.

- A textual description of the study equivalent in detail to a published methods section. For a checklist of which details should be included, see Poldrack et al. (2007).
- Copies of any stimulus files and programs used to administer the task.
- A description of all different analyses performed on the data, describing their purpose and outcome, and specific information about the location of any scripts used to run the analysis.
- Copies of any abstracts, presentations, or papers associated with the study.

B.4 Scripting for data analysis

The ability to script analyses is, in our opinion, essential to the ability to effectively analyze fMRI data. There are a number of advantages to using scripts as opposed to running analyses by hand. First, it can greatly increase the efficiency of analyses. Whereas it may be reasonable to run small numbers of analyses using a GUI-driven program, as the size of datasets increases it can become almost impossible to execute analyses manually. In addition, the use of scripts can make it much easier to try multiple different analyses, which can be important given the large number of arbitrary choices that one must make in setting up any particular analysis. Second, scripting can decrease the likelihood of errors, which are bound to occur when one manually specifies the details of an analysis. Third, scripting allows one to exactly reconstruct the details of any analysis, and rerun the analysis if necessary.

There are a number of scripting languages, and the choice of language is generally much less important than the decision to script in the first place, as most of them have similar capabilities from the standpoint of automating fMRI analysis. Some popular choices follow:

- UNIX Shell scripting languages, such as varieties of the Bourne shell (*sh*/*bash*) or C shell (*csh*/*tcsh*), in combination with the UNIX tools *sed* and *awk*
- Python
- PERL
- MATLAB

The choice of scripting language interacts with the particular software package being used; SPM users will likely choose MATLAB, whereas users of FSL or AFNI can use nearly any of the scripting languages described here.

An example.   Here we provide a simple example of what one can do using scripting with FSL. The files used for this example are available on the book Web site, as are a number of other scripts used for preprocessing and other operations.

We begin by using the FSL Feat GUI to set up the design for a single run for a single subject. This creates a set of design files, including design.fsf (which contains the description of the design), design.mat (which contains the design matrix), and design.con (which contains the contrasts). If the design is the same across subjects (i.e., contains the same conditions), then we can take advantage of the use of consistent naming schemes across subjects to create a new design file for each subject by replacing the relevant parts in the original file. The script below automatically creates and runs FSL analyses for multiple subjects using the design.fsf file (here called input.fsf) created for the first subject. Note that to use this successfully, all files that FSL expects (such as the onset files for each condition) must have the same name and be in the same relative location for each subject.

```
#!/bin/sh

BASEDIR="/path/to/data/directory"
ANALYSIS_NAME="analysis2_parametric"

doanalysis()
{
### IF THE DIRECTORY DOESN'T ALREADY EXIST, CREATE IT
if [ ! -e $BASEDIR/$SUB/analysis/analysis2_parametric ]
then
    mkdir $BASEDIR/$SUB/analysis/analysis2_parametric
fi

### CHANGE TO THE ANALYSIS DIRECTORY
cd $BASEDIR/$SUB/analysis/analysis2_parametric

### SET UP RUN 1
sed -e "s/SUB_001/${SUB}/" -e "s/EPI_4/EPI_$
{SCANS_INDEX[0]}/"
-e "s/S004_4D_mcf_brain.hdr/S00${SCANS_INDEX[0]}_4D_m
cf_brain.hdr/"
$BASEDIR/orig.fsf > $BASEDIR/$SUB/analysis/
$ANALYSIS_NAME/run1.fsf;


### SET UP RUN 2
sed -e "s/SUB_001/${SUB}/"  -e "s/EPI_4/EPI_$
{SCANS_INDEX[1]}/"
-e "s/S004_4D_mcf_brain.hdr/S00${SCANS_INDEX[1]}_4D_m
cf_brain.hdr/"
-e "s/run1/run2/" $BASEDIR/orig.fsf
> $BASEDIR/$SUB/analysis/$ANALYSIS_NAME/run2.fsf;


### EXECUTE FEAT FOR EACH RUN
```

```
for j in $DESIGN_NAME
do
    feat  $BASEDIR/$SUB/analysis/$ANALYSIS_NAME/$j
done

}


########### RUN ANALYSIS FOR SUBJECT 2
SUB="SUB_002"
DESIGN_NAME=("run1.fsf" "run2.fsf")
SCANS_INDEX=(4 5)
doanalysis


########### RUN ANALYSIS FOR SUBJECT 3
SUB="SUB_002"
DESIGN_NAME=("run1.fsf" "run2.fsf")
SCANS_INDEX=(5 7)
doanalysis
```

B.4.1 Some nuggets for scripting fMRI analyses

Here are some tips that may be useful when writing scripts for fMRI analysis.

- If creating file names that include numbers in them to represent an index, always use numbers that are zero-padded (e.g., "file0001.nii" rather than "file1.nii"). The reason for this is that the utilities that list file names (such as the UNIX *ls* command) do so alphabetically, which will result in misordering if used on files without zero-padding.

- It is often useful to first create a script that prints out all of the commands that it will execute, without actually executing them, to make sure that the correct commands will be executed.

- Always use absolute path names in scripts rather than relative path names.

- In general, avoid deleting files as part of a script. If files must be deleted, be sure to use absolute path names, and never use wild cards (e.g., *rm* *).

- For complex scripts, it is often useful to to write another script or program (e.g., using MATLAB or a scripting language) to create the script. Anytime one finds one's self doing the same operation many times by hand, it is likely that a script could help streamline the operation, prevent errors, and provide an enduring record of the operations that were performed.

Appendix C: Image formats

In the early days of fMRI, image formats were truly a Tower of Babel. Because most data were collected using research pulse sequences, the data were largely reconstructed offline and saved to file formats that varied from center to center. Because most analysis software was also written in-house, this was not a particular problem, so long as one didn't need to share data between centers. As the field developed, several standard file formats came into use, and the use of different formats between centers or laboratories was largely driven by the requirements of different analysis software packages, but until recently there still remained a substantial variety of file formats. Fortunately, the situation has gotten much better in the last decade, with the development and near-universal implementation of a common file format, known as *NiFTI*. In this appendix, we briefly describe some general issues regarding the storage of fMRI data along with some of the most important file formats.

C.1 Data storage

As discussed in Chapter 2, MRI data are usually stored in a binary data file as either 8- or 16-bit integers. The size of the data file on disk will thus be the product of the data size and the dimensions of the image. For example, storing a 16-bit integer image with dimensions of $128 \times 128 \times 96$ will take up 25,165,824 bits (or 3 megabytes). In addition to the raw image data, we also generally wish to store additional information about the image, which we refer to as *metadata*. These data describe various aspects of the image, such as the dimensions and the data type. This is important because it would not be possible to tell by looking at an binary dataset whether, for example, it was a $128 \times 128 \times 96$ image collected at 16 bits or a $128 \times 128 \times 192$ image collected at 8 bits. As discussed here, different image formats retain very different amounts and kinds of metadata.

Structural MRI images are generally stored as three-dimensional data files. Because fMRI data are collected as a series of images, they can be stored either as a set of three-dimensional files, or as a single four-dimensional file, where the

Table C.1. Description of some medical image data formats

Format Name	File Extension	Origin
Analyze	.img/.hdr	Analyze software, Mayo Clinic
DICOM	none	ACR/NEMA consortium
NIfTI	.nii or .img/.hdr	NIH Neuroimaging Informatics Tools Initiative
MINC	.mnc	Montreal Neurological Institute (extension of NetCDF)
AFNI brick	.BRIK	AFNI software, Medical College of Wisconsin/NIMH

fourth dimension is time. We generally prefer to store data as four-dimensional if possible, since it minimizes the number of files that must be dealt with, but some analysis packages cannot handle four-dimensional files.

C.2 File formats

Throughout the history of neuroimaging there has been a large number of different image formats; several of these are described in Table C.1. Here we describe the three most important formats at present: DICOM, Analyze, and NIfTI.

C.2.1 DICOM

Most MRI scanners today save their reconstructed data to a format called *DICOM*. This format arose from a consortium involving the American College of Radiologists (ACR) and the National Electronics Manufacturers Association (NEMA). DICOM is much more than simply an image storage format; it provides a protocol by which different imaging systems can communicate different forms of data, of which MRI images are one particular type. The current version of DICOM was introduced in 1993 and is supported by all of the major MRI scanner vendors.

DICOM generally stores each slice as a separate file; these files are conventially named using numbers reflecting the slice number, though this can vary between systems. The header information is embedded into the file and must be extracted using special software that can read and "dump" the header information. Of all of the different formats, DICOM retains the greatest amount of meta-data in the header, including low-level information about the scanner and image acquisition as well as information about the subject.

Although DICOM is the standard format for outputting data from MRI scanners, it is almost always necessary to convert from DICOM to some other format before data analysis. The main reason is that DICOM datasets are unwieldy, owing to the storage of each slice as a separate file. This can soon lead to massive numbers of small files that clog file systems and slow analysis. There are a number of freely available tools that can convert DICOM data files to any of the other major storage formats.[1]

---

[1] For some reason, there is a tendency for imaging researchers to try to develop their own conversion programs for file formats rather than using existing conversion software. In our opinion, this is a waste of time, in

C.2.1.1 Mosaic data storage

Some MRI pulse sequences (particularly on Siemens MRI systems) store fMRI datasets to DICOM as a *mosaic*, in which each image contains a mosaic of 16 actual slices presented as a single image. This is done to economize storage space, in cases where the scanner prefers to save images that have a dimension of 256×256, whereas fMRI images generally have a matrix size of 64×64. These mosaic images must generally be unpacked before analysis, in order to create three- or four-dimensional files that can be recognized by the analysis software.

C.2.2 Analyze

One of the best-known older formats for MRI data is known as Analyze; its name comes from a software package of the same name that was developed at the Mayo Clinic (and rarely used by fMRI researchers due to its expense). Analyze stores each dataset in a set of two files. A *data file*, which has the extension .img, contains the binary data for the image. A *header* file, which as the extension .hdr, contains the metadata for the image. Analyze was a popular format in the early days of fMRI, but it has largely been supplanted by the NIfTI format. Its main limitation is that the header has a relatively limited representation of the image metadata.

C.2.3 NIfTI

In 2000, the National Institute of Mental Health and the National Institute of Neurological Disorders and Stroke instituted a consortium of researchers to develop a new data storage format that would help alleviate problems with data sharing across different centers and software packages. In 2004, the first version of a new file format, known as NIfTI-1, was released. This format is an extension of the Analyze 7.5 format, adding a number of additional kinds of metadata. One of the most important features in the NIfTI format is a way to represent the relationship between voxel indices and spatial locations in the MRI scanner. When used properly, this helps to ensure that one can always accurately determine which direction is which (e.g., which side of the image represents the left side of the brain).

The standard file extension for NIfTI images is .nii, which contains both the header and image data. However, because of the relation between NIfTI and Analyze formats, it is also possible to represent NIfTI images using separate image (.img) and header (.hdr) files. One convenient feature of the single-file .nii format is that the files can be compressed using standard compression software (e.g., gzip), and some software packages (e.g., FSL) can directly read and write compressed .nii files (which have the extension .nii.gz).

---

addition to a potential source of errors. There are many unsolved problems in neuroimaging that are worthy of the attention of smart scientist/programmers, but conversion from DICOM to other standard image formats is not one of them.

Bibliography

Abdi, H. 2003. Partial least squares regression (PLS-regression), in *Encyclopedia for research methods for the social sciences*, M. Lewis Beck, A. Bryman, and T. Futing, Eds. Thousand Oaks, CA: Sage, 792–5.

Adler, R, & Taylor, J. 2007. *Random fields and geometry*. New York, NY: Springer.

Aguirre, GK, Zarahn, E & D'Esposito, M. 1997. Empirical analyses of BOLD fMRI statistics. II. Spatially smoothed data collected under null-hypothesis and experimental conditions. *Neuroimage*, 5, 199–212.

Aguirre, GK, Zarahn, E & D'Esposito, M. 1998. The inferential impact of global signal covariates in functional neuroimaging analyses. *Neuroimage*, 8(3), 302–6.

Alpaydin, E. 2004. *Introduction to machine learning*. Cambridge, Mass.: MIT Press.

Amunts, K, Schleicher, A, Bürgel, U, Mohlberg, H, Uylings, H B, & Zilles, K. 1999. Broca's region revisited: Cytoarchitecture and intersubject variability. *J Comp Neurol*, 412(2), 319–41.

Andersson, JL, Hutton, C, Ashburner, J, Turner, R, & Friston, K. 2001. Modeling geometric deformations in EPI time series. *Neuroimage*, 13(5), 903–19.

Ardekani, BA, Bachman, AH, Strother, SC, Fujibayashi, Y, & Yonekura, Y. 2004. Impact of inter-subject image registration on group analysis of fMRI data. *International Congress Series*, 1265, 49–59. Quantitation in Biomedical Imaging with PET and MRI. Proceedings of the International Workshop on Quantitation in Biomedical Imaging with PET and MRI.

Arnold, JB, Liow, JS, Schaper, KA, Stern, JJ, Sled, JG, Shattuck, DW, Worth, AJ, Cohen, MS, Leahy, RM, Mazziotta, JC, & Rottenberg, DA. 2001. Qualitative and quantitative evaluation of six algorithms for correcting intensity nonuniformity effects. *Neuroimage*, 13(5), 931–43.

Ashburner, J. 2007. A fast diffeomorphic image registration algorithm. *Neuroimage*, 38(1), 95–113.

Ashburner, J, & Friston, K. 2005. Unified segmentation. *Neuroimage*, 26(3), 839–51.

Ashburner, J, & Friston, KJ. 1999. Nonlinear spatial normalization using basis functions. *Hum Brain Mapp*, 7(4), 254–266.

Ashburner, J, & Friston, KJ. 2007. Non-linear registration, KJ Friston, J Ashburner, S Kiebel, TE Nichols, & Penny, WD (Eds)., In *Statistical parametric mapping: the analysis of functional brain images*, 1st ed, London: Elsevier/Academic Press.

Bassett, DS, & Bullmore, E. 2006. Small-world brain networks. *Neuroscientist*, 12(6), 512–23.

Beckmann, CF, & Smith, SM. 2004. Probabilistic independent component analysis for functional magnetic resonance imaging. *IEEE Trans Med Imaging*, 23(2), 137–52.

Beckmann, CF, & Smith, SM. 2005. Tensorial extensions of independent component analysis for multisubject FMRI analysis. *Neuroimage*, **25**(1), 294–311.

Bellman, RE. 1961. *Adaptive control processes*. Princeton, N.J.: Princeton University Press.

Benjamini, Y, & Hochberg, Y. 1995. Controlling the false discovery rate: a practical and powerful approach to multiple testing. *J R Stat Soc. Ser B Methodol*, **57**(1), 289–300.

Bentler, PM, & Stein, JA. 1992. Structural equation models in medical research. *Stat Methods Med Res*, **1**(2), 159–181.

Birn, RM, Diamond, JB, Smith, MA, & Bandettini, PA. 2006. Separating respiratory-variation-related fluctuations from neuronal-activity-related fluctuations in fMRI. *Neuroimage*, **31**, 1536–48.

Bishop, CM. 2006. *Pattern recognition and machine learning*. New York: Springer.

Biswal, B, Yetkin, FZ, Haughton, VM, & Hyde, JS. 1995. Functional connectivity in the motor cortex of resting human brain using echo-planar MRI. *Magn Reson Med*, **34**(4), 537–41.

Boesen, K, Rehm, K, Schaper, K, Stoltzner, S, Woods, R, Lüders, E, & Rottenberg, D. 2004. Quantitative comparison of four brain extraction algorithms. *Neuroimage*, **22**(3), 1255–61.

Bokde, AL, Tagamets, MA, Friedman, RB, & Horwitz, B. 2001. Functional interactions of the inferior frontal cortex during the processing of words and word-like stimuli. *Neuron*, **30**(2), 609–17.

Bollen, KA. 1989. *Structural equations with latent variables*. New York: Wiley.

Box, GE, Jenkins, GM, & Reinsel, GC. 2008. *Time series analysis: Forcasting and control*. Hoboken, NJ: John Wiley.

Boynton, GM, Engel, SA, Glover, GH, & Heeger, DJ. 1996. Linear systems analysis of functional magnetic resonance imaging in human V1. *J Neurosci*, **16**(13), 4207–21.

Bracewell, RN. 2000. *The Fourier transform and its applications*. 3rd ed. Boston: McGraw Hill.

Brett, M, Leff, AP, Rorden, C, & Ashburner, J. 2001. Spatial normalization of brain images with focal lesions using cost function masking. *Neuroimage*, **14**(2), 486–500.

Brett, M, Johnsrude, IS, & Owen, AM. 2002. The problem of functional localization in the human brain. *Nat Rev Neurosci*, **3**(3), 243–9.

Buckner, RL, Bandettini, PA, O'Craven, KM, Savoy, RL, Petersen, SE, Raichle, ME, & Rosen, BR. 1996. Detection of cortical activation during averaged single trials of a cognitive task using functional magnetic resonance imaging. *Proc Natl Acad Sci U S A*, **93**(25), 14878–83.

Buckner, RL, Head, D, Parker, J, Fotenos, AF, Marcus, D, Morris, JC, & Snyder, AZ. 2004. A unified approach for morphometric and functional data analysis in young, old, and demented adults using automated atlas-based head size normalization: Reliability and validation against manual measurement of total intracranial volume. *Neuroimage*, **23**(2), 724–38.

Bullmore, E, Horwitz, B, Honey, G, Brammer, M, Williams, S, & Sharma, T. 2000. How good is good enough in path analysis of fMRI data? *Neuroimage*, **11**(4), 289–301.

Bullmore, E, Long, C, Suckling, J, Fadili, J, Calvert, G., Zelaya, F, Carpenter, T.A, & Brammer, M. 2001. Colored noise and computational inference in neurophysiological (fMRI) time series analysis: Resampling methods in time and wavelet domains. *Hum Brain Mapp*, **12**(2), 61–78.

Bullmore, ET, Suckling, J, Overmeyer, S, Rabe-hesketh, S, Taylor, E, & Brammer, MJ. 1999. Global, voxel, and cluster tests, by theory and permutation, for a difference between two groups of structural MR images of the brain. *IEEE Trans. Med. Imaging*, **18**, 32–42.

Burgund, ED, Kang, HC, Kelly, JE, Buckner, RL, Snyder, AZ, Petersen, SE, & Schlaggar, BL. 2002. The feasibility of a common stereotactic space for children and adults in fMRI studies of development. *Neuroimage*, **17**(1), 184–200.

Buxton, RB. 2001. The elusive initial dip. *Neuroimage*, **13**(6 Pt 1), 953–8.

Buxton, RB, Wong, EC, & Frank, LR. 1998. Dynamics of blood flow and oxygenation changes during brain activation: the balloon model. *Magn Reson Med;* **39**(6), 855–64.

Buxton, RB. 2002. *Introduction to functional magnetic resonance imaging: Principles and techniques.* Cambridge, UK: Cambridge University Press.

Calhoun, VD, Liu, J, & Adali, T. 2009. A review of group ICA for fMRI data and ICA for joint inference of imaging, genetic, and ERP data. *Neuroimage*, **45**(1 Suppl), S163–72.

Cao, J, & Worsley, KJ. 2001. *Spatial statistics: Methodological Aspscts and Applications.* Lecture Notes in Statistics; vol. 159., New York: Springer, Chapter 8. Applications of random fields in human brain mapping, pp. 169–82.

Carmack, PS, Spence, J, Gunst, RF, Schucany, WR, Woodward, WA, & Haley, RW. 2004. Improved agreement between Talairach and MNI coordinate spaces in deep brain regions. *Neuroimage*, **22**(1), 367–71.

Caviness, Jr, VS, Kennedy, DN, Richelme, C, Rademacher, J, & Filipek, PA. 1996. The human brain age 7–11 years: A volumetric analysis based on magnetic resonance images. *Cereb Cortex*, **6**(5), 726–36.

Christensen, GE, Rabbitt, RD, & Miller, MI. 1994. 3D brain mapping using a deformable neuroanatomy. *Phys Med Biol*, **39**(3), 609–18.

Chumbley, JR, & Friston, KJ. 2009. False discovery rate revisited: FDR and topological inference using Gaussian random fields. *Neuroimage*, **44**(1), 62–70.

Clarke, LP, Velthuizen, RP, Camacho, MA, Heine, JJ, Vaidyanathan, M, Hall, LO, Thatcher, RW, & Silbiger, ML. 1995. MRI segmentation: Methods and applications. *Magn Reson Imaging*, **13**(3), 343–68.

Cleveland, WS. 1979. Robust locally weighted regression and smoothing scatterplots. *J Am Stat Assoc*, **74**, 829–836.

Cohen, AL, Fair, DA, Dosenbach, NU, Miezin, FM, Dierker, D, Van Essen, DC, Schlaggar, BL, & Petersen, SE 2008. Defining functional areas in individual human brains using resting functional connectivity MRI. *Neuroimage*, **41**, 45–57.

Cohen, J. 1988. *Power analysis for the behavioral sciences.* Hillsdale, NJ: Lawrence Erlbaum Associates.

Cohen, JR, Asarnow, RF, Sabb, FW, Bilder, RM, Bookheimer, SY, Knowlton, BJ, & Poldrack, RA. 2010. Decoding developmental differences and individual variability in response inhibition through predictive analyses across individuals. *Front Hum Neurosci*, **4**, 47.

Cohen, MS. 1997. Parametric analysis of fMRI data using linear systems methods. *Neuroimage*, **6**(2), 93–103.

Cohen, MS, & DuBois, RM. 1999. Stability, repeatability, and the expression of signal magnitude in functional magnetic resonance imaging. *J Magn Reson Imaging*, **10**(1), 33–40.

Cohen, MS, DuBois, RM, & Zeineh, MM. 2000. Rapid and effective correction of RF inhomogeneity for high field magnetic resonance imaging. *Hum Brain Mapp*, **10**(4), 204–11.

Cole, DM, Smith, SM, & Beckmann, CF. 2010. Advances and pitfalls in the analysis and interpretation of resting-state FMRI data. *Front Syst Neurosci*, **4**, 8.

Costafreda, SG. 2009. Pooling FMRI data: Meta-analysis, mega-analysis and multicenter studies. *Front Neuroinformat*, **3**, 33.

Dale, AM. 1999. Optimal experimental design for event-related fMRI. *Hum Brain Mapp*, **8**(2–3), 109–14.

Dale, AM, & Buckner, RL. 1997. Selective averaging of rapidly presentd individual trials using fMRI. *Hum Brain Mapp*, **5**, 329–340.

David, O, Guillemain, I, Saillet, S, Reyt, S, Deransart, C, Segebarth, C, & Depaulis, A. 2008. Identifying neural drivers with functional MRI: An electrophysiological validation. *PLoS Biol*, **6**(12), 2683–97.

Desai, R, Liebenthal, E, Possing, ET, Waldron, E, & Binder, JR. 2005. Volumetric vs. surface-based alignment for localization of auditory cortex activation. *Neuroimage*, **26**(4), 1019–29.

Desikan, RS, Ségonne, F, Fischl, B, Quinn, BT, Dickerson, BC, Blacker, D, Buckner, RL, Dale, AM, Maguire, RP, Hyman, BT, Albert, MS, & Killiany, RJ. 2006. An automated labeling system for subdividing the human cerebral cortex on MRI scans into gyral based regions of interest. *Neuroimage*, **31**(3), 968–80.

D'Esposito, M, Deouell, LY, & Gazzaley, A. 2003. Alterations in the BOLD fMRI signal with ageing and disease: A challenge for neuroimaging. *Nat Rev Neurosci*, **4**(11), 863–72.

Detre, JA, & Wang, J. 2002. Technical aspects and utility of fMRI using BOLD and ASL. *Clin Neurophysiol*, **113**(5), 621–34.

Devlin, JT, & Poldrack, RA. 2007. In praise of tedious anatomy. *Neuroimage*, **37**(4), 1033–41.

Duda, RO, Hart, PE, & Stork, DG. 2001. *Pattern classification*, 2nd ed. New York: Wiley.

Duvernoy, HM. 2005. *The human hippocampus: Functional anatomy, vascularization, and serial sections with MRI*, 3rd ed. Berlin: Springer.

Duvernoy, HM., & Bourgouin, P. 1999. *The human brain: Surface, three-dimensional sectional anatomy with MRI, and blood supply*, 2nd. ed. Wien: Springer.

Eickhoff, SB, Stephan, KE, Mohlberg, H, Grefkes, C, Fink, GR, Amunts, K, & Zilles, Karl. 2005. A new SPM toolbox for combining probabilistic cytoarchitectonic maps and functional imaging data. *Neuroimage*, **25**(4), 1325–35.

Ericsson, KA, Krampe, RT, & Tesch-Romer, C. 1993. The role of deliberate practice in the acquisition of expert performance. *Psychol Rev*, **100**, 363–406.

Evans, A, Collins, D, Mills, S, Brown, E, Kelly, R, & Peters, T. 1993. 3D statistical neuroanatomical models from 305 MRI volumes. *Nuclear Science Symposium and Medical Imaging Conference, 1993, 1993 IEEE Conference Record*, January. vol. 3, 1813–17.

Fair, DA, Dosenbach, NUF, Church, JA, Cohen, AL, Brahmbhatt, S, Miezin, FM, Barch, DM, Raichle, ME, Petersen, SE, & Schlaggar, BL. 2007. Development of distinct control networks through segregation and integration. *Proc Natl Acad Sci U S A*, **104**(33), 13507–12.

Fair, DA, Cohen, AL, Power, JD, Dosenbach, NUF, Church, JA, Miezin, FM, Schlaggar, BL, & Petersen, SE. 2009. Functional brain networks develop from a "local to distributed" organization. *PLoS Comput Biol*, **5**(5), e1000381.

Finger, S. 1994. *Origins of neuroscience: A history of explorations into brain function*. New York: Oxford University Press.

Fischl, B, Sereno, MI, Tootell, RB, & Dale, AM. 1999. High-resolution intersubject averaging and a coordinate system for the cortical surface. *Hum Brain Mapp*, **8**(4), 272–84.

Fischl, B, Salat, DH, Busa, E, Albert, M, Dieterich, M, Haselgrove, C, van der Kouwe, A, Killiany, R, Kennedy, D, Klaveness, S, Montillo, A, Makris, N, Rosen, B, & Dale, AM. 2002. Whole brain segmentation: Automated labeling of neuroanatomical structures in the human brain. *Neuron*, **33**(3), 341–55.

Forman, SD, Cohen, JD, Fitzgerald, JD, Eddy, WF, Mintun, MA, & Noll, DC. 1995. Improved assessment of significant activation in functional magnetic resonance imaging (fMRI): Use of a cluster-size threshold. *Magn Reson Med*, **33**, 636–47.

Fox, MD, Snyder, AZ, Vincent, JL, Corbetta, M., Van Essen, DC, & Raichle, ME. 2005. The human brain is intrinsically organized into dynamic, anticorrelated functional networks. *Proc Natl Acad Sci USA*, **102**, 9673–78.

Freire, L, & Mangin, JF. 2001. Motion correction algorithms may create spurious brain activations in the absence of subject motion. *Neuroimage*, **14**(3), 709–22.

Freire, L, Roche, A, & Mangin, JF. 2002. What is the best similarity measure for motion correction in fMRI time series? *IEEE Trans Med Imaging*, **21**(5), 470–84.

Friston, K. 1994. Functional and effective connectivity in neuroimaging: A synthesis. *Hum Brain mapp* **2**, 56–78.

Friston, KJ. 2005. Models of brain function in neuroimaging. *Annu Rev Psychol*, **56**, 57–87.

Friston, K, Jezzard, P, & Turner, R. 1994a. Analysis of functional MRI time-series. *Hum Brain Mapp*, **1**, 1–19.

Friston, KJ, Worsley, KJ, Frackowiak, RSJ, Mazziotta, JC, & Evans, AC. 1994b. Assessing the significance of focal activations using their spatial extent. *Hum Brain Mapp*, **1**, 210–20.

Friston, KJ, Frith, CD, Liddle, PF, & Frackowiak, RS. 1993. Functional connectivity: The principal-component analysis of large (PET) data sets. *J Cereb Blood Flow Metab*, **13**(1), 5–14.

Friston, KJ, Holmes, A, Poline, JB, Price, CJ, & Frith, CD. 1996a. Detecting activations in PET and fMRI: Levels of inference and power. *Neuroimage*, **4**(3), 223–35.

Friston, KJ, Williams, S, Howard, R, Frackowiak, RS, & Turner, R. 1996b. Movement-related effects in fMRI time-series. *Magn Reson Med*, **35**(3), 346–55.

Friston, KJ, Buechel, C, Fink, GR, Morris, J, Rolls, E, & Dolan, RJ. 1997. Psychophysiological and modulatory interactions in neuroimaging. *Neuroimage*, **6**(3), 218–29.

Friston, KJ, Fletcher, P, Josephs, O, Holmes, A, Rugg, MD, & Turner, R. 1998. Event-related fMRI: Characterizing differential responses. *Neuroimage*, **7**, 30–40.

Friston, KJ, Josephs, O, Zarahn, E, Holmes, AP, Rouquette, S, & Poline, J. 2000. To smooth or not to smooth? Bias and efficiency in fMRI time-series analysis. *Neuroimage*, **12**, 196–208.

Friston, KJ, Harrison, L, & Penny, W. 2003. Dynamic causal modelling. *Neuroimage*, **19**(4), 1273–302.

Friston, KJ, Penny, WD, & Glaser, DE. 2005. Conjunction revisited. *Neuroimage*, **25**(3), 661–7.

Friston, KJ, Rotshtein, P, Geng, JJ, Sterzer, P, & Henson, RN. 2006. A critique of functional localisers. *Neuroimage*, **30**(4), 1077–87.

Gavrilescu, M, Shaw, ME, Stuart, GW, Eckersley, P, Svalbe, ID, & Egan, GF. 2002. Simulation of the effects of global normalization procedures in functional MRI. *Neuroimage*, **17**, 532–42.

Genovese, CR, Lazar, NA, & Nichols, TE. 2002. Thresholding of statistical maps in functional neuroimaging using the false discovery rate. *Neuroimage*, **15**(4), 870–78.

Gitelman, DR, Penny, WD, Ashburner, J, & Friston, KJ. 2003. Modeling regional and psychophysiologic interactions in fMRI: the importance of hemodynamic deconvolution. *Neuroimage*, **19**(1), 200–7.

Glover, GH. 1999. Deconvolution of impulse response in event-related BOLD fMRI. *Neuroimage*, **9**(4), 416–29.

Glover, GH, Li, TQ, & Ress, D. 2000. Image-based method for retrospective correction of physiological motion effects in fMRI: RETROICOR. *Magn Reson Med*, **44**(1), 162–7.

Goutte, C, Nielsen, FA, & Hansen, LK. 2000. Modeling the haemodynamic response in fMRI using smooth FIR filters. *IEEE Trans Med Imaging*, **19**(12), 1188–201.

Graybill, FA. 1961. *An introduction to linear statistical models*. New York, NY: McGraw-Hill.

Greicius, MD, & Menon, V. 2004. Default-mode activity during a passive sensory task: Uncoupled from deactivation but impacting activation. *J Cogn Neurosci*, **16**, 1484–92.

Greicius, MD, Flores, BH, Menon, V, Glover, GH, Solvason, HB, Kenna, H, Reiss, AL, & Schatzberg, AF 2007. Resting-state functional connectivity in major depression: Abnormally increased contributions from subgenual cingulate cortex and thalamus. *Biol Psychiat*, **62**, 429–437.

Grinband, J, Wager, TD, Lindquist, M, Ferrera, VP, & Hirsch, J. 2008. Detection of time-varying signals in event-related fMRI designs. *Neuroimage*, **43**, 509–520.

Guimaraes, AR, Melcher, JR, Talavage, TM, Baker, JR, Ledden, P, Rosen, BR, Kiang, NY, Fullerton, BC, & Weisskoff, RM. 1998. Imaging subcortical auditory activity in humans. *Hum Brain Mapp*, **6**(1), 33–41.

Guo, Y, & Pagnoni, G. 2008. A unified framework for group independent component analysis for multi-subject fMRI data. *Neuroimage*, **42**(3), 1078–93.

Guyon, I, Weston, J, Barnhill, S, & Vapnik, V. 2002. Gene selection for cancer classification using support vector machines. *Machine Learning*, **46**(1–3), 389–422.

Hammers, A, Allom, R, Koepp, MJ, Free, SL, Myers, R, Lemieux, Louis, M, TN, Brooks, DJ, & Duncan, JS. 2003. Three-dimensional maximum probability atlas of the human brain, with particular reference to the temporal lobe. *Hum Brain Mapp*, **19**(4), 224–47.

Handwerker, DA, Ollinger, JM, & D'Esposito, M. 2004. Variation of BOLD hemodynamic responses across subjects and brain regions and their effects on statistical analyses. *Neuroimage*, **21**, 1639–1651.

Hanson, SJ, & Halchenko, YO. 2008. Brain reading using full brain support vector machines for object recognition: There is no "face" identification area. *Neural Comput*, **20**(2), 486–503.

Hanson, SJ, Matsuka, T, & Haxby, JV. 2004. Combinatorial codes in ventral temporal lobe for object recognition: Haxby (2001) revisited: is there a "face" area? *Neuroimage*, **23**(1), 156–66.

Harms, MP, & Melcher, JR. 2002. Sound repetition rate in the human auditory pathway: Representations in the waveshape and amplitude of fMRI activation. *J Neurophysiol*, **88**(3), 1433–50.

Harville, DA. 1997. *Matrix algebra from a statisticians perspective*. New York, NY: Springer Science and Buisness Medicine.

Hastie, T, Tibshirani, R, & Friedman, JH. 2001. *The elements of statistical learning: Data mining, inference, and prediction, with 200 full-color illustrations*. New York: Springer.

Hastie, T, Tibshirani, R, & Friedman, JH. 2009. *The elements of statistical learning: Data mining, inference, and prediction*, (2nd ed.). New York: Springer.

Haxby, JV, Gobbini, MI, Furey, ML, Ishai, A, Schouten, JL, & Pietrini, P. 2001. Distributed and overlapping representations of faces and objects in ventral temporal cortex. *Science*, **293**(5539), 2425–30.

Hayasaka, S, & Nichols, TE. 2003. Validating cluster size inference : Random field and permutation methods. *Neuroimage*, **20**, 2343–56.

Hayasaka, S, & Nichols, TE. 2004. Combining voxel intensity and cluster extent with permutation test framework. *Neuroimage*, **23**(1), 54–63.

Hayasaka, S, Peiffer, AM, Hugenschmidt, CE, & Laurienti, PJ. 2007. Power and sample size calculation for neuroimaging studies by non-central random field theory. *Neuroimage*, 37(3), 721–30.

Haynes, JD, & Rees, G. 2006. Decoding mental states from brain activity in humans. *Nat Rev Neurosci*, 7(7), 523–534.

Haynes, JD, Sakai, K, Rees, G, Gilbert, S, Frith, C, & Passingham, RE. 2007. Reading hidden intentions in the human brain. *Curr Biol*, 17(4), 323–28.

Henson, RNA, Buchel, C, Josephs, O, & Friston, KJ. 1999. The slice-timing problem in event-related fMRI. *NeuroImage*, 9, 125.

Henson, RNA, Shallice, T, Gorno-Tempini, ML, & Dolan, RJ. 2002. Face repetition effects in implicit and explicit memory tests as measured by fMRI. *Cerebral cortex*, 12(2), 178–86.

Hoenig, JM, & Heisey, DM. 2001. The abuse of power: The pervasive fallacy of power calculations for data analysis. *Amer Stat*, 55, 19–24.

Holden, M. 2008. A review of geometric transformations for nonrigid body registration. *IEEE Trans Med Imaging*, 27(1), 111–128.

Holmes, AP, & Friston, KJ. 1999. Generalisability, random effects & population inference. *Neuroimage*, 7(4 (2/3)), S754. *Proceedings of Fourth International Conference on Functional Mapping of the Human Brain*, June 7–12, 1998, Montreal, Canada.

Hutton, C, Bork, A, Josephs, O, Deichmann, R, Ashburner, J, & Turner, R. 2002. Image distortion correction in fMRI: A quantitative evaluation. *Neuroimage*, 16(1), 217–40.

Hyvärinen, A, & Oja, E. 2000. Independent component analysis: algorithms and applications. *Neural Networks*, 13(4-5), 411–30.

Jenkinson, M, & Smith, S. 2001. A global optimisation method for robust affine registration of brain images. *Med Image Anal*, 5(2), 143–56.

Jenkinson, M, Bannister, P, Brady, M, & Smith, S. 2002. Improved optimization for the robust and accurate linear registration and motion correction of brain images. *Neuroimage*, 17(2), 825–41.

Jezzard, P, & Balaban, RS. 1995. Correction for geometric distortion in echo planar images from B0 field variations. *Magn reson Med*, 34(1), 65–73.

Josephs, O, & Henson, RN. 1999. Event-related functional magnetic resonance imaging: Modelling, inference and optimization. *Philos Trans R Soc Lon. Ser. B Biol Sci*, 354(1387), 1215–28.

Josephs, O, Turner, R, & Friston, K. 1997. Event-related f MRI. *Hum Brain Mapp*, 5, 243–248.

Junghofer, M, Schupp, HT, Stark, R, & Vaitl, D. 2005. Neuroimaging of Emotion: empirical effects of proportional global signal scaling in fMRI data analysis. *Neuroimage*, 25, 520–6.

Kao, M-H, Mandal, A, Lazar, N, & Stufken, J. 2009. Multi-objective optimal experimental designs for event-related fMRI studies. *Neuroimage*, 44(3), 849–56.

Klein, A, Andersson, J, Ardekani, BA, Ashburner, J, Avants, B, Chiang, M-C, Christensen, GE, Collins, DL, Gee, J, Hellier, P, Song, JH, Jenkinson, M, Lepage, C, Rueckert, D, Thompson, P, Vercauteren, T, Woods, RP, Mann, JJ, & Parsey, RV. 2009. Evaluation of 14 nonlinear deformation algorithms applied to human brain MRI registration. *Neuroimage*, 46(3), 786–802.

Kohavi, R. 1995. A Study of cross-validation and bootstrap for accuracy estimation and model selection. *International Joint Conference on Artificial Intelligence*. San Francisco, CA: Morgan Kaufmann Publishers, 1137–43.

Kriegeskorte, N, Goebel, R, & Bandettini, P. 2006. Information-based functional brain mapping. *Proc Natl Acad Sci U S A*, 103(10), 3863–8.

Kriegeskorte, N, Simmons, WK, Bellgowan, PSF, & Baker, CI. 2009. Circular analysis in systems neuroscience: The dangers of double dipping. *Nat Neurosci*, **12**(5), 535–40.

Kruggel, F., & von Cramon, DY. 1999. Temporal properties of the hemodynamic response in functional MRI. *Hum Brain Mapp*, **8**, 259–71.

Kwong, KK, Belliveau, JW, Chesler, DA, Goldberg, IE, Weisskoff, RM, Poncelet, BP, Kennedy, DN, Hoppel, BE, Cohen, MS, & Turner, R. 1992. Dynamic magnetic resonance imaging of human brain activity during primary sensory stimulation. *Proc Natl Acad Sci U S A*, **89**(12), 5675–9.

Lancaster, JL, Woldorff, MG, Parsons, LM, Liotti, M, Freitas, CS, Rainey, L, Kochunov, PV, Nickerson, D, Mikiten, SA, & Fox, PT. 2000. Automated Talairach atlas labels for functional brain mapping. *Hum Brain Mapp*, **10**(3), 120–31.

Lancaster, JL, Tordesillas-Gutiérrez, D, Martinez, M, Salinas, F, Evans, A, Zilles, K, Mazziotta, JC, & Fox, PT. 2007. Bias between MNI and Talairach coordinates analyzed using the ICBM-152 brain template. *Hum Brain Mapp*, **28**(11), 1194–205.

Lange, N, & Zeger, S. 1997. Non-linear Fourier time series analysis for human brain mapping by functional magnetic resonance imaging. *Appl Statistics*, **46**, 1–29.

Lindquist, MA, & Wager, TD. 2007. Validity and power in hemodynamic response modeling: a comparison study and a new approach. *Hum Brain Mapp*, **28**(8), 764–84.

Liu, T. 2004. Efficiency, power, and entropy in event-related fMRI with multiple trial types. Part II: Design of experiments. *Neuro Image*, **21**(1), 401–13.

Liu, T, & Frank, LR. 2004. Efficiency, power, and entropy in event-related FMRI with multiple trial types. Part I: Theory. *Neuroimage*, **21**(1), 387–400.

Liu, TT, Frank, LR, Wong, EC, & Buxton, RB 2001. Detection power, estimation efficiency, and predictability in event-related fMRI. *Neuroimage*, **13**, 759–73.

Logothetis, NK, Pauls, J, Augath, M, Trinath, T, & Oeltermann, A. 2001. Neurophysiological investigation of the basis of the fMRI signal. *Nature*, **412**, 150–7.

Lucerna, S, Salpietro, FM, Alafaci, C, & Tomasello, F. 2004. *In vivo atlas of deep brain structures*. Berlin Heidelberg, Germany: Springer.

Mai, JK, Assheuer, J, & Paxinos, G. 2004. *Atlas of the human brain, (2nd ed.)* San Diego: Academic Press.

Mandeville, B, Marota, JJ, Ayata, C, Zaharchuk, G, Moskowitz, MA, Rosen, BR, & Weisskoff, RM. 1999. Evidence of a cerebrovascular postarteriole windkessel with delayed compliance. *J Cereb Blood Flow Metab*, **19**(6), 679–89.

Marcus, DS, Wang, TH, Parker, J, Csernansky, JG, Morris, JC, & Buckner, RL. 2007. Open access series of imaging studies (OASIS): Cross-sectional MRI data in young, middle aged, nondemented, and demented older adults. *J Cogn Neurosci*, **19**(9), 1498–507.

McIntosh, AR. 1999. Mapping cognition to the brain through neural interactions. *Memory*, **7**(5–6), 523–48.

McIntosh, AR. 2000. Towards a network theory of cognition. *Neural Netw*, **13**(8–9), 861–70.

McIntosh, AR, Bookstein, FL, Haxby, JV, & Grady, CL. 1996. Spatial pattern analysis of functional brain images using partial least squares. *Neuroimage*, **3**(3–1), 143–57.

McIntosh, AR, & Lobaugh, NJ. 2004. Partial least squares analysis of neuroimaging data: Applications and advances. *Neuroimage*, **23 Suppl 1**, S250–63.

Miezin, FM, Maccotta, L, Ollinger, JM, Petersen, SE, & Buckner, RL. 2000. Characterizing the hemodynamic response: effects of presentation rate, sampling procedure, and the possibility of ordering brain activity based on relative timing. *Neuroimage*, **11**(6–1), 735–59.

Miller, MI. 2004. Computational anatomy: Shape, growth, and atrophy comparison via diffeomorphisms. *Neuroimage*, **23 Suppl 1**, S19–33.

Moody, J, McFarland, DA, & Bender-deMoll, S. 2005. Visualizing network dynamics. *Amer J Sociol*, **110**, 1206–41.

Mori, S, Wakana, S, & Van Zijl, PCM. 2004. *MRI atlas of human white matter*. 1st ed. Amsterdam: Elsevier.

Mourão-Miranda, J, Friston, KJ, & Brammer, M. 2007. Dynamic discrimination analysis: A spatial-temporal SVM. *Neuroimage*, **36**(1), 88–99.

Mumford, JA, & Nichols, TE. 2008. Power calculation for group fMRI studies accounting for arbitrary design and temporal autocorrelation. *Neuroimage*, **39**(1), 261–8.

Mumford, JA, & Nichols, T. 2009. Simple group fMRI modeling and inference. *Neuroimage*, **47**(4), 1469–75.

Muresan, L, Renken, R, Roerdink, JBTM, & Duifhuis, H. 2005. Automated correction of spin-history related motion artefacts in fMRI: simulated and phantom data. *IEEE transactions on bio-medical engineering*, **52**(8), 1450–60.

Murphy, K, Birn, RM, Handwerker, DA, Jones, TB, & Bandettini, PA. 2009. The impact of global signal regression on resting state correlations: are anti-correlated networks introduced? *Neuroimage*, **44**, 893–905.

Neter, J, Kutner, M, Wasserman, W, & Nachtshiem, C. 1996. *Applied linear statistical models*. McGraw-Hill Irwin.

Newman, MEJ. 2003. The structure and function of complex networks. *SIAM Rev*, **45**(2), 167–256.

Newman, MEJ, Barabási, A-L, & Watts, DJ. 2006. *The structure and dynamics of networks*. Princeton: Princeton University Press.

Nichols, TE, & Holmes, Andrew P. 2002. Nonparametric permutation tests for functional neuroimaging: a primer with examples. *Hum Brain Mapp*, **15**(1), 1–25.

Nichols, TE, & Hayasaka, S. 2003. Controlling the familywise error rate in functional neuroimaging: A comparative review. *Stat Meth Med Res*, **12**(5), 419–446.

Nichols, T, Brett, Matthew, A, Jesper, Wager, Tor, & Poline, J.B. 2005. Valid conjunction inference with the minimum statistic. *Neuroimage*, **25**(3), 653–60.

Nieto-Castanon, A, Ghosh, SS, Tourville, JA, & Guenther, FH. 2003. Region of interest based analysis of functional imaging data. *Neuroimage*, **19**(4), 1303–16.

Norman, KA, Polyn, SM, Detre, GJ, & Haxby, JV. 2006. Beyond mind-reading: Multi-voxel pattern analysis of fMRI data. *Trends Cogn Sci*, **10**(9), 424–30.

Oakes, TR, Johnstone, T, Walsh, KSO, Greischar, LL, Alexander, AL, Fox, AS, & Davidson, RJ. 2005. Comparison of fMRI motion correction software tools. *Neuroimage*, **28**(3), 529–43.

Orban, GA, & Vanduffel, W. 2007. Comment on Devlin and Poldrack. *Neuroimage*, **37**(4), 1057–8; discussion 1066–8.

Ostuni, JL, Santha, AK, Mattay, VS, Weinberger, DR, Levin, RL, & Frank, JA. 1997. Analysis of interpolation effects in the reslicing of functional MR images. *J Comput Assist Tomog*, **21**(5), 803–10.

O'Toole, AJ, Jiang, F, Abdi, H, Penard, N, Dunlop, JP, & Parent, MA. 2007. Theoretical, statistical, and practical perspectives on pattern-based classification approaches to the analysis of functional neuroimaging data. *J Cogn Neurosci*, **19**(11), 1735–52.

Pearl, J. 2000. *Causality: Models, reasoning, and inference*. Cambridge: Cambridge University Press.

Penhune, VB, Zatorre, RJ, MacDonald, D, and Evans, AE. 1996. Interhemispheric anatomical differences in human primary auditory cortex: Probabilistic mapping and volume measurement from MR scans. *Cerebral Cortex*, 6(5), 661–672.

Penny, WD, Stephan, KE, Mechelli, A, & Friston, KJ. 2004. Modelling functional integration: A comparison of structural equation and dynamic causal models. *Neuroimage*, 23 **Suppl** 1, S264–74.

Pluim, J, Maintz, J, & Viergever, M. 2003. Mutual-information-based registration of medical images: A survey. *Med Imaging* 22(8), 986–1004.

Poldrack, RA. 2007. Region of interest analysis for fMRI. *Soc Cogn Affect Neurosci*, 2(1), 67–70.

Poldrack, RA, Fletcher, PC, Henson, RN, Worsley, KJ, Brett, M, & Nichols, TE. 2007. Guidelines for reporting an fMRI study. *Neuroimage* 40(2), 409–14.

Poldrack, RA, Halchenko, YO, & Hanson, SJ. 2009. Decoding the large-scale structure of brain function by classifying mental states across individuals. *Psychol Sci* 20(11), 1364–72.

Poline, JB, & Mazoyer, BM. 1993. Analysis of individual positron emission tomography activation maps by detection of high signal-to-noise-ratio pixel clusters. *J Cereb Blood Flow Metabol*, 13(3), 425–37.

Posner, MI, Petersen, SE, Fox, PT, & Raichle, ME. 1988. Localization of cognitive operations in the human brain. *Science*, 240(4859), 1627–31.

Postelnicu, G, Zollei, L, & Fischl, B. 2009. Combined volumetric and surface registration. *IEEE Trans Med Imaging*, 28(4), 508–22.

Press, WH. 2007. *Numerical recipes: The art of scientific computing*, 3rd ed. Cambridge: Cambridge University Press.

Protzner, AB, & McIntosh, AR. 2006. Testing effective connectivity changes with structural equation modeling: What does a bad model tell us? *Hum Brain Mapp*, 27(12), 935–47.

Rademacher, J, Morosan, P, Schormann, T, Schleicher, A, Werner, C, Freund, HJ, et al. (2001). Probabilistic mapping and volume measurement of human primary auditory cortex. *Neuroimage*, 13(4), 669–683.

Raichle, ME, MacLeod, AM, Snyder, AZ, Powers, WJ, Gusnard, DA, & Shulman, GL. 2001. A default mode of brain function. *Proc Natl Acad Sci U S A*, 98(2), 676–82.

Ramsey, JD, Hanson, SJ, Hanson, C, Halchenko, YO, Poldrack, RA, & Glymour, C. 2010. Six problems for causal inference from fMRI. *Neuroimage*, 49(2), 1545–58.

Ravasz, E, Somera, AL, Mongru, DA, Oltvai, ZN, & Barabási, AL. 2002. Hierarchical organization of modularity in metabolic networks. *Science*, 297(5586), 1551–5.

Rissman, J, Gazzaley, A, & D'Esposito, M. 2004. Measuring functional connectivity during distinct stages of a cognitive task. *Neuroimage*, 23(2), 752–63.

Rizk-Jackson, A, Mumford, J, & Poldrack, RA. 2008. Classification analysis of rapid event-related fMRI studies. *Org Hum Brain Mapp Abst*.

Roche, A, Malandain, G, Pennec, X, & Ayache, N. 1998. The correlation ratio as a new similarity measure for multimodal image registration. *Proc MICCAI*, January.

Roebroeck, A, Formisano, E, & Goebel, R. 2005. Mapping directed influence over the brain using Granger causality and fMRI. *Neuroimage*, 25(1), 230–42.

Rowe, JB, Hughes, LE, Barker, RA, & Owen, AM. 2010. Dynamic causal modelling of effective connectivity from fMRI: Are results reproducible and sensitive to Parkinson's disease and its treatment? *Neuroimage*, 52(3), 1015–26.

Samanez-Larkin, GR, & D'Esposito, M. 2008. Group comparisons: Imaging the aging brain. *Soc Cogn Affect Neurosci*, **3**(3), 290–7.

Schmahmann, JD. 2000. *MRI atlas of the human cerebellum*. San Diego: Academic Press.

Schmithorst, VJ, & Holland, SK. 2004. Comparison of three methods for generating group statistical inferences from independent component analysis of functional magnetic resonance imaging data. *J Magn Reson Imaging*, **19**(3), 365–8.

Shallice, T. 1988. *From neuropsychology to mental structure*. Cambridge: Cambridge University Press.

Shattuck, DW, Sandor-Leahy, SR, Schaper, KA, Rottenberg, DA, & Leahy, RM. 2001. Magnetic resonance image tissue classification using a partial volume model. *Neuroimage*, **13**(5), 856–76.

Shattuck, DW, Mirza, M, Adisetiyo, V, Hojatkashani, C, Salamon, G, Narr, KL, Poldrack, RA, Bilder, RM, & Toga, AW. 2008. Construction of a 3D probabilistic atlas of human cortical structures. *Neuroimage*, **39**(3), 1064–80.

Shipley, B. 2000. *Cause and correlation in biology: A user's guide to path analysis, structural equations, and causal inference*. Cambridge: Cambridge University Press.

Shmuel, A, & Leopold, DA. 2008. Neuronal correlates of spontaneous fluctuations in fMRI signals in monkey visual cortex: Implications for functional connectivity at rest. *Hum Brain Mapp*, **29**, 751–61.

Shulman, GL, Fiez, JA, Corbetta, M, Buckner, RL, Miezin, FM, Raichle, ME, & Petersen, SE. 1997. Common blood flow changes across visual tasks: II. Decreases in cerebral cortex. *J Cogn Neurosci*, **9**(5), 648–63.

Sled, J, & Pike, G. 1998. Understanding intensity nonuniformity in MRI. *Proc. Med Image Comput Computer-Assisted Intervention*, **1496**, 614–22.

Sled, JG, Zijdenbos, AP, & Evans, AC. 1998. A nonparametric method for automatic correction of intensity nonuniformity in MRI data. *IEEE Trans Med Imaging*, **17**(1), 87–97.

Smith, AM, Lewis, BK, Ruttimann, UE, Ye, FQ, Sinnwell, TM, Yang, Y, Duyn, JH, & Frank, JA. 1999. Investigation of low frequency drift in fMRI signal. *Neuroimage*, **9**, 526–33.

Smith, SM, & Nichols, TE. 2009. Threshold-free cluster enhancement: Addressing problems of smoothing, threshold dependence and localisation in cluster inference. *Neuroimage*, **44**(1), 83–98.

Smith, SM, Fox, PT, Miller, KL, Glahn, DC, Fox, PM, Mackay, CE, Filippini, N, Watkins, KE, Toro, R, Laird, AR, & Beckmann, CF. 2009. Correspondence of the brain's functional architecture during activation and rest. *Proc Natl Acad Sci U S A*, **106**(31), 13040–5.

Spirtes, P, Glymour, CN, & Scheines, R. 2000. *Causation, prediction, and search*, 2nd ed. Cambridge, Mass.: MIT Press.

Sporns, O, Chialvo, DR, Kaiser, M, & Hilgetag, CC. 2004. Organization, development and function of complex brain networks. *Trends Cogn Sci (Regul Ed)*, **8**(9), 418–25.

Stephan, KE, Hilgetag, CC, Burns, GA, O'Neill, MA, Young, MP, & Kötter, R. 2000. Computational analysis of functional connectivity between areas of primate cerebral cortex. *Philos Trans R Soc Lond B Biol Sci*, **355**(1393), 111–26.

Stephan, KE, Weiskopf, N, Drysdale, PM, Robinson, PA, & Friston, KJ. 2007. Comparing hemodynamic models with DCM. *Neuroimage*, **38**(3), 387–401.

Stephan, KE, Kasper, L, Harrison, LM, Daunizeau, J, den Ouden, H EM, Breakspear, M, & Friston, KJ. 2008. Nonlinear dynamic causal models for fMRI. *Neuroimage*, **42**(2), 649–62.

Stephan, KE, Penny, WD, Moran, RJ, den Ouden, HEM, Daunizeau, J, & Friston, KJ. 2010. Ten simple rules for dynamic causal modeling. *Neuroimage*, **49**(4), 3099–109.

Studholme, C, Hill, D, & Hawkes, D. 1999. An overlap invariant entropy measure of 3D medical image alignment. *Pattern Recog.* **32**, 71–86.

Swanson, N, & Granger, C. 1996. Impulse response functions based on a causal approach to residual orthogonalization in vector autoregressions. *J Amer. Stat Assoc*, **92**, 357–67.

Talairach, J. 1967. *Atlas d'anatomie stéréotaxique du télencéphale: études anatomo-radiologiques.* Paris: Masson et Cie.

Talairach, J, & Tournoux, P. 1988. *Co-planar stereotaxic atlas of the human brain.* Stuttgart: Thieme.

Thesen, S, Heid, O, Mueller, E, & Schad, LR. 2000. Prospective acquisition correction for head motion with image-based tracking for real-time fMRI. *Magn Reson Med*, **44**(3), 457–65.

Thevenaz, P, Blu, T, & Unser, M. 2000. Interpolation revisited. *IEEE Trans Med Imaging*, **19**(7), 739–58.

Toga, AW, & Thompson, PM. 2001. Maps of the brain. *Anat Rec*, **265**(2), 37–53.

Toga, AW, & Thompson, PM. 2005. Genetics of brain structure and intelligence. *Annu Rev Neurosci*, **28**, 1–23.

Tohka, J, Foerde, K, Aron, AR, Tom, SM, Toga, AW, & Poldrack, RA. 2008. Automatic independent component labeling for artifact removal in fMRI. *Neuroimage*, **39**(3), 1227–45.

Tom, SM, Fox, CR, Trepel, C, & Poldrack, RA. 2007. The neural basis of loss aversion in decision-making under risk. *Science*, **315**(5811), 515–18.

Translational College of LEX. 1997. *Who is Fourier?: A mathematical adventure*, 2nd ed. Boston: Language Research Foundation.

Troendle, JF, Korn, EL, & McShane, LM. 2004. An example of slow convergence of the bootstrap in high dimensions. *American Statistician*, **58**(1), 25–9.

Tzourio-Mazoyer, N, Landeau, B, Papathanassiou, D, Crivello, F, Etard, O, Delcroix, N, Mazoyer, B, & Joliot, M. 2002. Automated anatomical labeling of activations in SPM using a macroscopic anatomical parcellation of the MNI MRI single-subject brain. *Neuroimage*, **15**(1), 273–89.

Uylings, HBM, Rajkowska, G, Sanz-Arigita, E, Amunts, K, & Zilles, K. 2005. Consequences of large interindividual variability for human brain atlases: Converging macroscopical imaging and microscopical neuroanatomy. *Anat Embryol (Berl)*, **210**(5–6), 423–31.

Van Essen, DC. 2005. A Population-Average, Landmark- and surface-based (PALS) atlas of human cerebral cortex. *Neuroimage*, **28**(3), 635–62.

Van Essen, DC, & Dierker, D. 2007. On navigating the human cerebral cortex: Response to "in praise of tedious anatomy". *Neuroimage*, **37**(4), 1050–4; discussion 1066–8.

Vazquez, a L, & Noll, DC. 1998. Nonlinear aspects of the BOLD response in functional MRI. *Neuroimage*, **7**(2), 108–18.

Vul, E, Harris, C, Winkielman, P, & Pashler, H. 2009. Puzzlingly high correlations in fMRI Studies of emotion, personality, and social cognition. *Perspect Psychol Sci*, **4**, 274–90.

Wager, TD, & Nichols, TE. 2003. Optimization of experimental design in fMRI: A general framework using a genetic algorithm. *Neuroimage*, **18**(2), 293–309.

Wager, TD, Vazquez, A, Hernandez, L, & Noll, DC. 2005. Accounting for nonlinear BOLD effects in fMRI: Parameter estimates and a model for prediction in rapid event-related studies. *Neuroimage*, **25**(1), 206–18.

Watts, DJ. 2003. *Six degrees: The science of a connected age*, 1st ed. New York: Norton.

Weissenbacher, A, Kasess, C., Gerstl, F, Lanzenberger, R, Moser, E, & Windischberger, C. 2009. Correlations and anticorrelations in resting-state functional connectivity MRI: A quantitative comparison of preprocessing strategies. *Neuroimage*, **47**, 1408–16.

Wilke, M, Schmithorst, VJ, & Holland, SK. 2002. Assessment of spatial normalization of whole-brain magnetic resonance images in children. *Hum Brain Mapp*, **17**(1), 48–60.

Woods, R, Mazziotta, J, & Cherry, S. 1993. MRI-PET registration with automated algorithm. *J Comput Assist Tomogr* **17**(4), 536–46.

Woolrich, MW, Behrens, TEJ, & Smith, SM. 2004a. Constrained linear basis sets for HRF modelling using variational Bayes. *Neuroimage*, **21**(4), 1748–61.

Woolrich, MW, Behrens, TEJ, Beckmann, CF, Jenkinson, M, & Smith, SM. 2004b. Multilevel linear modelling for FMRI group analysis using Bayesian inference. *Neuroimage*, **21**(4), 1732–47.

Woolrich, MW, Ripley, BD, Brady, M, & Smith, SM. 2001. Temporal autocorrelation in univariate linear modeling of FMRI data. *Neuroimage*, **14**(6), 1370–86.

Woolsey, TA, Hanaway, J, & Gado, MH. 2008. *The brain atlas: A visual guide to the human central nervous system*, 3rd ed. Hoboken, N.J.: Wiley.

Worsley, KJ, Liao, CH, Aston, J, Petre, V, Duncan, GH, Morales, F, & Evans, AC. 2002. A general statistical analysis for fMRI data. *Neuroimage*, **15**, 1–15.

Wu, D H, Lewin, J S, & Duerk, J L. 1997. Inadequacy of motion correction algorithms in functional MRI: Role of susceptibility-induced artifacts. *J Magn Reson Imaging*, **7**(2), 365–70.

Xue, G, Aron, AR, & Poldrack, RA. 2008. Common neural substrates for inhibition of spoken and manual responses. *Cereb Cortex*, **18**(8), 1923–32.

Yeşilyurt, B, Uğurbil, K, & Uludağ, K. 2008. Dynamics and nonlinearities of the BOLD response at very short stimulus durations. *Magn Reson Imaging*, **26**(7), 853–62.

Zarahn, E, Aguirre, GK, & D'Esposito, M. 1997. Empirical analyses of BOLD fMRI statistics. I. Spatially unsmoothed data collected under null-hypothesis conditions. *Neuroimage*, **5**, 179–97.

Zhang, B, & Horvath, S. 2005. A general framework for weighted gene co-expression network analysis. *Stat Appl Genet Mol Biol*, **4**, Article17.

Zhang, H, Nichols, TE, & Johnson, TD. 2009. Cluster mass inference via random field theory. *Neuroimage*, **44**(1), 51–61.

Zola-Morgan, S. 1995. Localization of brain function: The legacy of Franz Joseph Gall (1758-1828). *Annu Rev Neurosci*, **18**, 359–83.

Index

AC, *see* anterior commissure
AC-PC line, 54
aliasing, 49, 50
alternative hypothesis, 110
anatomical variability, 53–54
anterior commissure, 54
AR(1) + white noise model, 91
artifacts, 35
autoregressive moving average model, 91

balloon model, 153
basis function, 21, 31, 77
    constrained basis set, 79–81
Bayesian inference, 153
Bayesian statistics, 111
beta-series correlation, 133–134, 163
between-modality registration, 22
bias field correction, 56
Bonferroni, 122
Bonferroni correction, 117
bounding box, 54
brain extraction, 56–57
Brodmann's area, 178, 181–182

circularity, 116, 184
classifier, 161, 167–172
    assessing accuracy, 171
    characterizing, 171–172
    linear, 167
    nonlinear, 167
    sensitivity analysis, 171–172
cluster forming threshold, 114, 115
computational anatomy, 61
conditional independence, 150
conjuncion inference, *see* statistical inference;
        conjunction
connectivity
    effective, 144–155
    functional, 131–144
convolution, 32–74
coordinate space, 54
coordinate system, 15–16
coregistration, 60

cost function, 18, 21–26
    correlation ratio, 25–26
    least squares, 22–23
    mutual information, 23–25, 46
    normalized correlation, 23
cost function masking, 69
cross-validation, 165, 171
curse of dimensionality, 161

data organization, 202–204
deconvolution, 75, 133, 135, 136
default mode, 140, 159
design optimization, 98–99
diffeomorphism, 61
dimensionality reduction, 161, 167
directed graph, 145
discrete cosine transform basis, 88
dispersion derivative, 77
distortion correction, 38–41
drift, 6, 86
dropout, 38, 39
Duvernoy atlas, 178
dynamic causal model, 152–154

efficiency, 95–98
entropy, 23

false discovery rate, 121–123
familywise error rate, 117–121
FDR, *see* false discovery rate
feature selection, 161, 164–167
file format
    Analyze, 209–210
    BRIK, 209
    DICOM, 209
    MINC, 209
    NIfTi, 63, 208–210
filter
    high-pass, 32, 33, 88
    low-pass, 32, 33, 92
finite impulse response model, 77–80, 98, 186
FIR, *see* finite impulse response model

fixed effects model, 6, 104
fMRI
    event-related, 5, 133
    resting-state, 140
format
    numeric, 13–15
Fourier analysis, 31
Fourier transform, *see* Fourier analysis
Friston, Karl, 8
full width at half maximum, 51, 118
functional localization, 130
functional localizer, 185
functional specialization, 130
FWE, *see* familywise error rate

Gauss Markov theorem, 193
Gaussian random field theory, *see* random
        field theory
general linear model, 6, 103, 191–200
    estimation, 191
    multiple linear regression, 193
    simple linear regression, 192
    weighted linear regression, 196
geometric distortion, 38
ghosting, 35, 36
glass brain, *see* maximum intensity projection
GLM, *see* general linear model
global signal covariate, 158
Granger causality, 154–155
Granger causality mapping, 154
graph theory, 155
graphical causal model, 150–152
grid computing, 202

hemodynamic response, 2, 71–77, 133, 186
    assuming a shape, 79
    canonical, 75–77
    linearity, 6, 73–74, 187
    temporal resolution, 81–82
homogenous coordinates, 20
HRF, *see* hemodynamic response

ICA, *see* independent components analysis
independent components analysis, 37–38, 44, 50,
        138–143, 159, 167
inference, *see* statistical inference
interleaved acquisition, 41
interpolation, 18, 28–31, 46
    higher-order, 29–31
    linear, 29, 47
    nearest neighbor, 28–29
    sinc, 29–30, 47

jitter, 97
joint histogram, 24, 25

Lagrangian multiplier, 149
linear discriminant analysis, 170
LOWESS, 88

M-sequence, 98
machine learning, 6, 160
masking, *see* statistical inference; masking
maximum intensity projection, 175
metadata, 14, 208
mixed effects model, 6, 100–104
    between subject variance, 100
    compared to fixed effects model, 100–102
    ordinary least squares, 104
    two stage approach, 102–104
    within subject variance, 100
modeling
    ANOVA, 199
    contrasts, 194
    design matrix setup, 197–200
    interactions, 109
    mean centering covariates, 105–108
    motion parameters, 84
    paired *t*-test, 197
    response time, 82–84
    t-test, 197
mosaic data storage, 210
motion correction, 43–50
    interactions with slice timing correction, 48
    interactions with susceptibility, 47–48
    prospective, 47
    quality control for, 47
multifiducial mapping, 175
multiple testing problem, 116
multiscale optimization, 27
multivoxel pattern analysis, 6, 163
MVPA, *see* multivoxel pattern analysis, *see*
        multivoxel pattern analysis

NaN, *see* not a number
network analysis, 155–159
    preprocessing for, 157–159
neurological convention, 16
noise, 86–92
    1/f, 86
normalization
    children, 67–68
    choosing a method, 63–64
    data with lesions, 68, 69
    elderly, 68
    landmark-based, 60
    quality control, 65–66
    special populations, 66–68
    surface-based, 62–63, 175
    troubleshooting, 66–67
    volume-based, 60, 175
not a number, 59
nuisance model, 133, 157–158
null hypothesis, 110

operating systems, 202
orthogonal sections, 174
orthogonalization, 84
overfitting, 170, 161–170

P-value, 110
parametric modulation, 82

parametric simulations, 119
partial least squares, 143–144
path analysis, *see* structural equation modeling
pattern information analysis, *see* multivoxel pattern
    analysis
PC, *see* posterior commissure
PCA, *see* principal components analysis
percent signal change, 186–189
peristimulus time averaging, *see* selective averaging
PET, *see* positron emission tomography
phrenology, 130
physiological motion, 49
PLS, *see* partial least squares
positron emission tomography, 4
posterior commissure, 54
power, 111
power analysis, 126–129
    post hoc, 129
    ROI-based calculation, 127
power spectrum, 31, 32
PPI, *see* psychophysiological interaction
precoloring, 92
prewhitening, 90–91, 196
principal components analysis, 132, 137–138, 167
probabilistic atlas, 179, 182
processing stream, 10, 35, 58–60
project management, 204–205
psychophysiological interaction, 134–136, 158–159

quadratic discriminant analysis, 167
quality control, 34–38
quantization error, 15

radiological convention, 16
Raichle, Marcus, 140
RAID, 202
random field theory, 51, 114, 117–119
rank deficient, 194
recursive feature elimination, 167
region of interest, 116, 164, 183–189
    for inference, 126
registration
    landmark-based, 55
    linear, 63–64
    nonlinear, 63–64
regularization, 26–27
RESEL, 118
ROI, *see* region of interest

scripting, 205–207
searchlight procedure, 172
seed correlation, 131–133
selective averaging, 75
SEM, *see* structural equation modeling
skull stripping, *see* brain extraction
slice timing correction, 41–42
small volume correction, 126, 183
small-world network, 155–156
software package, 7
    AFNI, 8–9, 25, 60, 202
        alphasim, 119
        group modeling, 105
    AIR, 23, 26, 27

ART, 64
BFC, 57
Brain Voyager, 8, 9
CARET, 62, 175–177
choosing, 10
DARTEL, 61, 64
FastICA, 142
FreeSurfer, 9, 62, 63, 176, 179
FSL, 8–9, 23, 25–28, 58–60, 88, 91, 115,
        143, 202, 205
    FIRST, 179
    FLIRT, 64
    FLOBS, 79, 80
    FNIRT, 61, 62, 64
    FSLView, 65, 174
    group modeling, 105
    MELODIC, 141
    randomise, 120
GIFT, 143
IRTK, 64
MATLAB, 205
mricron, 175
PERL, 205
PyMVPA, 170
Python, 205
R, 170
SPM, 8, 25–27, 57–59, 77, 91, 132, 176, 202, 205
    group modeling, 105
    SnPM, 121
SYN, 64
TETRAD, 150–153
UNIX, 205
XNAT, 204
spatial smoothing, 50–52
spatiotemporal classifier, 163
spikes, 35, 36
spin history, 43
statistical inference
    Bayesian, 111–112
    classical, 110–112
    cluster mass, 114
    cluster size, 114
    cluster-level, 112–115
    conjunction, 125
    conjunctions, 126
    masking, 125
    nonparametric, 119–121
    set-level, 112, 115–116
    voxel-level, 112–113
statistical learning, *see* machine learning
stimulus correlated motion, 44
stimulus-driven transients, 131
structural equation modeling, 146–149, 154
support vector machine, 164, 170

Talairach atlas, 55, 177–178
Talairach space, 17, 54, 179–181
Talairach, Jean, 17, 19, 54
template
    custom, 68
    ICBM-152, 56
    MNI, 55, 60, 178, 181
temporal derivative, 77

TFCE, *see* threshold free cluster enhancement
threshold free cluster enhancement, 115
tissue segmentation, 57–58
transform
  affine, 18–19, 60
  discrete cosine, 21
  linear, 18, 19
  nonlinear, 19–21
  piecewise linear, 19
  rigid body, 19
Type I error, 111
Type II error, 111

unified segmentation, 58
UNIX, 202, 203

voodoo correlations, *see* circularity
voxel, 13
voxel-counting, 185

within-modality registration, 22
Woods criterion, 26